AF738438

GROUP PSYCHOTHERAPY
The Psychoanalytic Approach

Other titles by S. H. Foulkes
Introduction to Group Analytic Psychotherapy
Therapeutic Group Analysis
Group Analytic Psychotherapy: Methods and Principles
Selected Papers: Psychoanalysis and Group Analysis

Of related interest
David Rosenfeld: Psychoanalysis and Groups—History and Dialectics

GROUP PSYCHOTHERAPY

THE PSYCHOANALTYIC APPROACH

Second Edition

S.H. Foulkes & E.J. Anthony

Routledge
Taylor & Francis Group
LONDON AND NEW YORK

First published in 1957
Published 1984 by H. Karnac (Books) Ltd.

Published 2019 by Routledge
2 Park Square, Milton Park, Abingdon, Oxon OX14 4RN
605 Third Avenue, New York, NY 10017

First issued in hardback 2019

Routledge is an imprint of the Taylor & Francis Group, an informa business

Copyright © 1984 by Elizabeth Foulkes and E.J. Anthony

All rights reserved. No part of this book may be reprinted or reproduced or utilised in any form or by any electronic, mechanical, or other means, now known or hereafter invented, including photocopying and recording, or in any information storage or retrieval system, without permission in writing from the publishers.

Notice:
Product or corporate names may be trademarks or registered trademarks, and are used only for identification and explanation without intent to infringe.

British Library Cataloguing in Publication Data
A C.I.P. for this book is available from the British Library

ISBN 13: 978-0-367-09948-0 (hbk)
ISBN 13: 978-0-946439-10-2 (pbk)

Contents

We are grateful to Messrs Hamish Hamilton Ltd, the author, and the translator, for permission to use a short scene from Jean-Paul Sartre's *In Camera*.

Editorial Foreword

This book contains the first attempt to give a comprehensive account for the lay reader of the principles and methods of Group Psychotherapy – i.e. the treatment in groups of individuals suffering from indispositions of the mind. Nowadays the principles of individual psychotherapy, or psychoanalysis and related methods, are matters of fairly general knowledge. Information concerning group psychotherapy is scattered among papers in journals and books not easily accessible to, or not written for, the general reader.

Dr Foulkes and Dr Anthony have here collaborated not only to outline the relevant theory, but also to illuminate the subject with realistic case material. Naturally they have presented the subject from their own point of view, and even if this is distinctive it is representative of important trends in therapeutic theory and practice. The basic ideas are in fact extremely simple and not a matter of dispute among the major psychotherapeutic schools. It would appear to be a well authenticated fact that in merely bringing to mind and giving expression to repressed emotions and desires the patient may experience great relief and sometimes be restored to equanimity.

In this, indeed, there is nothing at all surprising. We have always heard that 'confession is good for the soul'. We have often encouraged those in distress 'to have a good cry', and those who are worried 'to get things off their chest'. We have all met cases of friends who after a violent quarrel were better friends than they ever were before. So familiar are these facts that we might well be tempted to accept an early theory, officially sponsored under the concept of 'abreaction', that the cause of all mental ills is 'repression' and the cure the removal of inhibitions.

This, however, all authorities now agree is an over-simplification. Two further matters, at least, require elucidation. First, how and why do some desires become so deeply repressed, and how can this buried material be brought back to the surface? Second, these repressed desires are found to derive from relations to persons (parents and siblings) and the 'abreaction' of the repression would seem to require a working off of emotion in relation to persons. The elucidation of the first of these matters leads to a complex theory of personality development, and the elucidation of the second to the complex and still unsettled theory of 'the transference'. In individual psychotherapy the recovery of buried material and the working through of stages of the transference are determined by the relations of the individual patient and the individual analyst. In group psychotherapy the process takes place within the setting of a group of half a dozen or so patients and an analyst acting in the role of the 'participant observer'. As free association is the basic technique of individual analysis, so 'free floating discussion' (as described in this book) is the basic technique of group therapy.

Literally uninhibited conversation is a phenomenon not to be found in nature, nor in any ordinary society. The quite spontaneous expression of whatever passes through the mind is restricted to rare and peculiar states and occasions such as, for example, extreme intoxication. Normally the thoughts that men express are carefully selected with due regard to conventions, customs, and taboos. Men, in general, in their conversation do not wish to wound or offend; and in addition they are concerned not to offend in order to save their own ego-encapsulating skins. They do not open up a conversation by expressing their adverse first impression of each other's personal appearance, nor do they discuss their necrophilic impulses with the freedom with which they describe their more refined gastronomic tastes – except in group psychotherapeutic sessions.

What happens when the normal inhibitions are removed? What then determines the content of conversation and what are the effects of conversations of this kind?

What happens, as might be expected, is that there are turns of conversation of a kind which may well occasion the raising of some eyebrows. Why precisely these turns should occur, and how these turns are connected with the deeper sources of anxiety and suffering, and what the effects may be that ensue upon the relaxation of inhibitions, it is the purpose of this book to explain.

Editorial Foreword

In the study of its authors' argument, the reader may properly feel that he is keeping abreast with one of the latest developments in psychotherapy, and that he is doing so at the growing point of a very difficult art and the growing point of a puzzling branch of science.

C. A. MACE

Chapter 1

Group Psychotherapy and Group-Analysis: Basic Considerations

1. INTRODUCTION

Group psychotherapy is now practised in clinics and institutions as well as in private practice all over the world. Beyond this there is a growing realization of its significance for other groups, social life in general, social psychiatry, community therapy, selection procedures and education.

There are many varieties and types of group psychotherapy. For a broad orientation it may be useful to consider these types according to whether their impact is primarily due to:

(*a*) *relief* through expression. Catharsis (action methods and activities of all sorts);
(*b*) *restoration* through participation and acceptance, best known as *encounter* groups; or in addition to these
(*c*) the *liberation* of creative forces in the individual, the *liquidation* of old fixations in development by laying bare disturbing conflicts, bringing them to awareness and resolution (group-analysis).

Only this last category, characteristic for the analytic approach, concerns us here. All the pioneers in this field came from psychoanalysis: T. Burrow, S. H. Foulkes, P. Schilder, S. R. Slavson, L. Wender and others. All of them were American, except S. H. Foulkes whose work developed independently in England. Only the latter, while always remaining a Freudian psychoanalyst in the individual field, maintained from the beginning that in this new field the group situation changes the therapeutic process decisively. Accordingly, he created a novel method of approach which he called group-analytic psychotherapy and new theoretical concepts: group-analysis. This view has more recently gained much ground. It is nevertheless fair to say that it is even now insufficiently understood and that psychoanalysts are more reluctant to accept the changes in method and theory involved than are other workers in this field.

The reader will find at the end of this book (p. 271) a selection of books from the vast literature which now exists on this subject. Some of the most important books we have included give a general survey and an integrated view from the early beginnings to the present time. Books which have a special merit for those interested in historical developments are also included. For the most part the reading list gives different analytical approaches with representatives from the different schools as they will presently be reviewed. Books which put more emphasis on research are also included. We also mention some of the more important journals in this field.

2. THE PSYCHO-ANALYTIC APPROACH

Let us now turn to the psychoanalytic approach to psychotherapy. We consider psychoanalysis as a therapeutic method taking place between two people, the analyst and his patient, and consider group-analysis as a form of psychotherapy and not as a form of psychoanalysis. We use the terms 'group-analysis' and 'group-analytic situation' as the equivalents, in a group situation, of 'psychoanalysis' and 'psychoanalytic situation'. If we wish to make explicit that we talk of group-analysis as a form of treatment, we use the term 'group-analytic psychotherapy'. This indicates that this method is analytic but primarily based on the group. It should however be understood that the analysis of the individual remains a primary concern. The individual is being treated *in the context* of the group with the active participation of the group. For a detailed description of this method, the reader is referred to S. H. Foulkes: *Therapeutic Group Analysis* (Allen & Unwin, 1964). A new comprehensive book on the method by the same author will soon appear.

Like other work which is considered in this book, we take as our starting point the practice and theory of psychoanalysis. The present writers stand firmly on the grounds of classical psychoanalysis whilst many other workers appear to have been trained within schools which, for short, one might call neo-Freudian. All these neo-analytic schools are not so much distinguished by what they have added to or developed from Freud's work, but by what they have left out or distorted. The foundation on which their approach to groups has been built up thus differs considerably. Nevertheless the same workers often refer to their practice as 'psychoanalysis' in groups. In truth they often violate psychoanalytic concepts whether in the individual or the group setting and consequently fail to do justice to the significant features of the group situation. The present writers consider that psychoanalytical concepts, clinical and theoretical, are firmly rooted to begin with in the one- and later in the two-personal situation. There is no intrinsic reason why psychoanalysis should not in future extend its dimension and claim that group-analysis is psychoanalysis in the multi-personal situation. If and when this should be stated it would become clear, however, that the whole of psychoanalytic theory and practice would have to be changed, and far removed from the mind and intention of its originator. For the time being, we think as psychoanalysts that this discipline has an important function to fulfil on its own grounds. We do no wish to inaugurate yet another neo-analytic school of thought.

In the meantime we firmly reject the idea that experiences in group psychotherapy should be limited by present-day psychoanalytical concepts. Group-analysis is free to develop within the larger framework of psychotherapy. Its effects inside this have been described as a revolution.

3. THE MAIN TRENDS

The first point we have to keep in mind when we consider the meaning and delineation which several authors give to an analytic approach is that their concept as to what is psychoanalysis differs significantly. Having this in mind, the main trends discernible at this point in time may be stated as follows (as they are stated briefly and summarily it will be appreciated that this account is over-simplified):

(*a*) If the psychotherapist is individually trained and experienced in psychoanalysis he will, and must, use psychoanalytical concepts to guide his practical actions. He will note that the group situation modifies all processes and introduces some new factors. The theory, which remains that of psychoanalysis, has to take note of these modifications. What we are dealing with is *analytic group psychotherapy* as represented most clearly in the work of S. R. Slavson. We agree with him in so far as psychoanalysis is concerned. We think that he takes psychoanalytical concepts too much as absolute truths, instead of relatively correct in their own setting, as perhaps all truth is. The more relevant difference between this view and the group-analytic position, however, concerns the valuation of the group situation and its influence on practice and theory.

(*b*) Psychoanalysis in the group is possible. The emphasis is on the individual in the group. Group dynamics do exist, but have no bearing on the ongoing treatment, group or no group. This view is held by A. Wolf who has been one of its pioneers and has considerably influenced the practice of 'psychoanalytic' group therapy in the U.S.A. In their book, *Psychoanalysis in Groups*, A. Wolf and E. K. Schwartz present a comprehensive and valuable account of their experiences, method and theories as practised at the Postgraduate Center for Mental Health in New York. Workers adhering to this view use to good effect the possibilities inherent in the stimulation and potentialities of a multipersonal interactive setting, and they feel, with us, that therapy is more effective and intensive in this setting than is the treatment of the isolated individual. To some extent their experience precludes them from understanding our views, as they work in a different situation in which they cannot well test and correct our premises. Their groups are large, up to ten members. Wolf and Schwartz prepare their patients by individual analysis, who may return to individual sessions if they become too anxious, though this is rarely necessary for prolonged periods. They have also worked with 'alternate sessions' taking place without the therapist's presence. There is no question that good psychotherapy can be done in this way, but the present writer, who independently had occasionally used similar procedures, found possible gains to be heavily outweighed by the advantages of analysing all conflicts in *one* single, clearly defined, therapeutic situation at one and the same period of time. Otherwise one works in a transference situation which is unnecessarily complicated. Schwartz and Wolf seem to make no allowances for this or the consequences concerning the theory of group dynamics. By this term we mean the psychodynamics in the group situation, which build up into an interconnected, transactional network.

(*c*) A third view which also originated in England, in particular at the Tavistock Clinic, is that the psychoanalyst follows exactly the same principles in the group as he does in the individual situation. The difference is that the whole group is now considered as if it were one patient. Thus a one-to-one relationship is restored, corresponding to the situation in individual psychoanalysis. The analyst confines himself to the interpretation of the transference situation as it presents itself in the ongoing session. This, in the 'here and now', is the centre of the procedure. Though these workers base their approach purely on psychoanalysis they have, like the present writers, refrained from calling it group psychoanalysis. This approach to groups was introduced by W. R. Bion (see Selected Reading list). The type of psychoanalysis on which it is based is strongly influenced by the theories of M. Klein and W. R. Fairbairn, in particular the so-called 'inner object' theory. This is really valid only on narcissistic, psychotic levels of mentality and Bion has indeed paid particular attention to these levels in his interpretations. Later followers, H. Ezriel amongst others, concern themselves exclusively with transference interpretation, reminiscent of James Strachey's conviction that these alone are effective, 'mutative'. For a critique of this work see S. Scheidlinger, *Group Process in Group Psychotherapy* I and II,* and also I. D. Yalom (see Selected Reading). Recently a concise account of this school of thought, edited by H. Walton, has appeared (see Selected Reading). This approach might be said to represent (psycho-) analysis of the group as a whole by the therapist. The main difference between this and the group-analytic position appears to lie in the much greater variety of interpretations used by us, and in a different view as to their dynamic significance. The active participation of the group itself is in our view much more important for psychotherapy in the group. At the same time, the function of the group as a whole has in our view a more primary significance for the understanding of all part processes concerning its members, and not the other way round ('trans-personal processes').

* *American Journal of Psychotherapy*, vol. XIV, no. 1, January 1960.

(*d*) The 'group-dynamic theory' originated by K. Lewin has influenced group psychotherapy in various ways. A certain cross-fertilization also took place between the Tavistock Institute of Human Relations in London and some American institutions influenced by him. Though this theory has no common ground with psychoanalysis, it seemed at first compatible with an analytic approach, as exemplified at the time by the work of G. R. Bach and C. Rogers.

This type of 'encounter' group clearly falls into our category (*b*): restoration through participation and acceptance (see p. 15). In recent years the term 'encounter' group has been extended to group activities with an emphasis on action. These may take their inspiration partly from Moreno's 'psychodrama', but go far beyond this as in communal bathing and other pursuits at Esalen, California. These are popular, sensational entertainments and do not claim to be psychotherapy. They appear to make an impression on the participants, sometimes to the good, sometimes to the bad. At best they may be regarded as helping the *anomie* of the isolated human individual estranged as he is from his community in the western culture. The openly anti-analytic bias of these methods has helped in bringing the analytical schools of group psychotherapy closer together.

We do not find that 'group dynamics' enter much into the small therapeutic group, and in this respect agree with Wolf and others. If occasionally we use terms which are also used in K. Lewin's work, they have a different connotation or dimension, though they need not necessarily clash with his usage. For our orientation to the hospital 'therapeutic community' at Northfield, we found that our own group-analytic views married well with concepts used in 'field theory', and that the latter helped us in our orientation. Here belongs for instance the concept of a social 'field'. Further, there is a common background as regards Gestalt psychology.

The present writer learned to appreciate the holist view of the human organism and all its consequences from his teacher K. Goldstein, and through his studies with Adhémar Gelb became convinced of the dictum that the whole is prior and more elementary than its parts. He considers the figure-ground relationship is of principal significance. As applied to group-analysis this is, however, extended in depth and applied to complex processes of interaction between the more obvious manifestations and their more silent or concealed background. Without the elucidation of this background they cannot be fully understood or even observed. Taking a very simple example: if a person leaves the group, this must be understood from that person's point of view as well as that of the rest of the group, and is in fact a result of their interaction.

The term 'group dynamics' has sometimes been used by us for 'group psychodynamics' in the sense of Freud's unconscious dynamics. In order to avoid confusion we later adopted instead the term '*group processes*'. As we shall presently make clear, to us intra-psychic does *not* convey, as to G. Bach, 'intradermic', and we look upon the dynamic processes in the group not from the outside, but from inside, as intra-psychic dynamics in their interaction.

4. THE GROUP-ANALYTIC VIEW

The group-analytic view itself is in the centre of this whole book and need not be set out here specifically. Some of it has been made clear in the preceding discussion of other approaches. A comprehensive and integrated presentation of this work in the preceding twenty-five years appeared in 1964.*

In spite of many and important differences there seems to be enough agreement between group-analysts – including ourselves – to set them apart from other non-analytic group psychotherapists, and for them to be considered as speaking the same language. Agreement largely exists with respect to the analytic attitude of the therapist, the guiding principles of his interventions, his concern with the dynamic unconscious, and the interpretation of resistances, defence reactions, transference, etc.

The importance of human experience, of the encounter, is also common ground among group-analysts, and probably all group psychotherapists. This element has been recently stressed by 'existential analysts' in individual as well as in group psychotherapy.

The most important issue between the different forms of analytic group psychotherapy is the varying significance attached to the

* S. H. Foulkes, op. cit.

group situation itself. It is in this respect that *group analysis* as understood by us takes a different position, both in practice and theory, by placing the group and the group situation decidedly in the centre.

The treatment of a patient within a group setting is so far removed from the psychoanalytic set-up – one could almost say it is its opposite – that in the writers' opinion it is misleading to call it psychoanalysis. In so far as the therapist is a psychoanalyst he will still be a psychoanalyst; one cannot be a psychoanalyst in the morning when sitting behind a couch and something else when sitting in a group in the afternoon. The patient too remains the same person, and what is true for him from a psychoanalytical point of view must still be true for him when he sits in a circle, as has been said long ago.* Such treatment is therefore psychotherapy of a psychoanalytical orientation.

It is, however, *group* psychotherapy. Psychoanalysis is principally biological and genetic in its approach. It views complex behaviour as motivated in the last resort by elementary instinctual drives which are firmly rooted in somatic needs. The ego is fundamentally a body-ego, says Freud. Only the therapeutic function of psychoanalysis brought social, interpersonal dynamics into orbit with the discovery of transference in the two-personal situation.

These interpersonal psychodynamics have a greater bearing on the *therapeutic* processes. Group psychotherapy which intensifies and amplifies the social, interactional aspects of psychodynamics is thus the situation of choice for the study of therapeutic and pathogenic processes as they operate in the immediate present, the here and now of the therapeutic situation.

The group situation is not a psychoanalytical situation *manquée*; it introduces powerful and completely new parameters of its own. These will be set forth throughout this book. Thus all experiences and theories in the wide field of the group psychotherapies, however far removed from an analytic approach, have common ground with our approach in view of their concern with people – patients or otherwise – in groups. It looks also as if people from all the different schools can make a new start and find common ground

* See S. H. Foulkes: *Introduction to Group Analytic Psychotherapy*, Heinemann, 1948.

in the observation of groups which they can share. As far as group-analytic psychotherapy is concerned it can therefore open its doors wide to all schools, however divergent their techniques and theories are in the individual field, particularly if they share an analytic background in the broader sense.

5. BASIC CONCEPTS OF GROUP PSYCHOTHERAPY

In the light of our own comprehensive group-analytic view we may now state some of the fundamental concepts of all group psychotherapy.

Human living has always been in groups. These are ever-changing according to conditions – geographical, economic, historical, technical, cultural. Correspondingly, the idea which the human individual has of himself and his group and of the relation between the two is ever-changing too.

In recent times, since the end of the Renaissance, and in a community which stresses individual property and competition, a configuration has arisen which created the idea of an individual person as if existing in isolation. He is then confronted with the community, the world, as if they were outside him. The philosophy of Descartes starts from this premise and its strict subject-object juxtaposition is still responsible for many pseudo problems of our time.* Yet one of the surest observations one can make is that the individual is preconditioned to the core by his community even before he is born, and imprinted vitally by the group which brings him up. This concerns even his genetic inheritance, and still more his psychology, in so far as this is developed in the interaction between him, objects and persons. The present writer's insight into this deep-going interrelationship between the individual and his group or community was stimulated by his close contact with sociologists such as the late Franz Borkenau and particularly also his intimate exchange of ideas over many years with Norbert Elias. Contributions from social anthropologists such as B. K. Malinowski, Margaret Mead, Meyer Fortes and others were, however, of even greater importance as no work on small groups existed in sociology at the time.

* See 'Queries on Existential Psychotherapy' by Marvin J. Feldman, *International Journal of Social Psychiatry*, vol. IX, no. 2, Spring 1963.

Group Psychotherapy

Nature itself speaks with a clear language. Throughout all species it is abundantly clear that the individual specimen is entirely unimportant and that the only thing which matters is the survival of the group, of the community. Modern circumstances tend also to conceive, and treat, the individual as expendable. Plans are made discounting literally millions of human lives without hesitation. No wonder the modern individual is afraid of the group – is afraid of losing his very existence, of his identity being submerged and submitted to the group. The individual, while helplessly compressed into a mere particle of social groups and masses, is at the same time left without any true companionship in regard to his inner mental life.

The relative isolation, alienation, of the individual is thus a very real problem of our time. Whereas all sickness is liable to register in this way, mental sickness has a disturbance of integration within the community at its very roots – a disturbance of communication. This modern sickness, so often displayed in deep doubts and fear about integrity and identity, is also reflected in our theoretical terms. Any mention of group dynamics gives rise to passionate objections by some of our theoreticians. They behave as if the individual was in mortal danger, awaiting their chivalrous championship for rescue.

To look upon any natural group as if it was the result of a confluence of isolated individuals is untenable. Paradoxically our own particular groups are really constructed of isolated strange individuals meeting for the purpose of treatment. Yet behind this strangeness are certain pre-conditions – often silently made – of which the most general ones are as follows:

(1) That the biological species is the same.

(2) That the cultural background is similar, which means among other things that there is agreement as to what is desirable normal behaviour: what is sick, good, bad, and so forth.

(3) That the patient and therapist speak the same language, literally as well as metaphorically – otherwise there cannot be an efficient communication between them.

(4) That the patient has reasons to lay himself open to the therapeutic process, his motivation.

(5) That we have a method of access to unconscious processes.

The last two points, 4 and 5, indicate why there is a premium on psychopathology; because it does appear that without disturbance, without pathology, these conditions are not fulfilled.

(6) That the relationship which develops on the basis of strong emotions is accepted and responded to in a particular fashion, expressed in a particular attitude and situation (the therapeutic situation).

(7) That the doctor at least takes into account the whole patient in the whole situation, though as a background. In the foreground are individual details as they are presented by the patient.

For our present purposes we are concerned only with groups in their psychological aspects, with psyche groups, to use Helen Jenning's term. We are further leaving out of account here the psychological relationship between groups, or between any particular group and the community of which it is a part, i.e. group dynamics. We are concerned with internal psychological processes, endo-psychic reality, intra-psychic mechanisms or dynamics. It is at this point that one is up against a prejudice deeply engrained, erroneous as it is.

6. GROUP AND INDIVIDUAL IN NEW PERSPECTIVE

We have become used to thinking of intra-psychic processes, *ipso facto* as inside the same individual person, inside the same skull as it were. If we make such an assumption we beg one of the most important questions which arises. The fact that these mental processes are taking place physically in each individual brain is undoubted. If we hear an orchestra playing a piece of music, all the individual noises are produced each on one particular individual instrument; yet what we hear is the orchestra playing music, the conductor's interpretation, etc. Not even in terms of pure sound do we hear a simple summary, a summation of all the individual waves which reach our ears, but these are modified significantly, being part and parcel of a total sound. In truth what we hear is the orchestra. In the same way mental processes going on in a group under observation reach us in the first place as a concerted whole. Those familiar with Gestalt psychology will find no difficulty in understanding that the whole is more elementary than the parts. With this insight we have arrived at one of the basic concepts in group psychotherapy without which all other observations are misinterpreted or insufficiently described, namely that what we experience in the first place is the *group as a whole*.

The network of all individual mental processes, the psychological medium in which they meet, communicate, and interact, can be called the *matrix*. This is of course a construct – in the same way as is for example the concept of traffic, or for that matter of mind. In further formulation of our observations we have come to conceive these processes not merely as interpersonal but as *transpersonal*. In short we have a concert of interactions which is our primary basis for orientation, for interpretation, confrontation, and other contributions. This orientation shows on which level our interventions are most useful, but the whole process is taking place solely for the benefit of the individual member. There can be no question of a problem of group versus individual, or individual versus group. These are two aspects, two sides of the same coin.

Psychoanalysis has shown that neuroses are based on conflict, conflict that arose early in life in relation to parents or their equivalents. This conflict, at bottom, is one between the individual's instinctive impulses and his group's cultural taboos. This becomes internalized, unconscious, in the dynamic and the systematic sense, that is to say subject to the operation of the primary process – primitive prelogical mentality. As soon as the therapist enters into the situation this endo-psychic material becomes capable of involving two persons. Even to call this interpersonal is not enough. It is an endo-psychic common union between two people. The analyst can afford to enter into the patient's primary world without having to respond from his own primary world. This is his particular contribution. Out of this common ground arises a relationship which becomes the battlefield for the solution of the patient's neurosis – the so-called transference neurosis. There is no need for us, nor do we wish, to abandon these foundations. Concepts like the Oedipus complex, patriarchal and matriarchal, assume a conflict based on the primary family group. Infantile sexuality, incest barriers, are all based on the species and its cultural development. Even fathers and mothers are archetypes, the personal father and mother only representing them. The culture and values of a community are inescapably transferred to the growing infant by its individual father and mother as determined by their particular nation, class, religion, and region. They are transmitted verbally or non-verbally, instinctively, and emotionally twenty-four hours a day and night. Even the objects, movements, gestures, and accents are determined in this way by these representatives of the cultural group. On top of this, but all permeating, is the particular individual personal stamp of the individual father and mother. Individual psychotherapy is thus a form of group psychotherapy without being aware of this.

Group psychotherapy only brings back the problems where they belong. The community is represented in the treatment room. Valuations and norms are re-stated and modified by comparison, contrast, and analysis. Communication leading to a shared experience and understanding is in terms of the group.

Group psychotherapy can be practised with or without an analytical orientation. In either case it operates in a group situation which it must take into account. Group-analytic method and theory do away with pseudo problems such as biological versus cultural, somatogenic versus psychogenic, individual versus group, reality versus phantasy. Instead we endeavour to use concepts which from the beginning do justice to an integrated view.

The first and foremost aspect with which group psychotherapists are usually concerned, and according to which they form their concepts, is that of belonging, of participation. Being a respected and effective member of the group, being accepted, being able to share, to participate, belong to the basic constructive experiences in human life. No health is conceivable without this. This happens throughout life, but the need for psychotherapy arises when this participation and sharing are disturbed. It is important because we have now to deal with the restoration of this disturbed communication. Resistances displayed within the group's interactional network or matrix reflect the unconscious defences within the individual. At this point it must be remembered that what is dynamically unconscious is also at the same time subject to the primary process. It belongs to the system *ucs* (unconscious), that is to say it is cast in a primitive symbolic language. This language is understood unconsciously, and transmission – communication – does take place without consciousness. The group, through processes of progressive communication, works its way through from this primary, symbolic level of expression into a conscious, articulate language. This *work in communication* is the operational basis of all therapy in the group. This leads us to the interpretative, psychoanalytic part of our work, which is superimposed on the constructive part of group participation, going hand in hand with it.

Group analysis as we understand it works on the group model. The processes which we know from a two-personal situation can be seen in full in interaction between two, three, and more persons. They can be seen as what they are: as *interactional processes*, not as processes in the isolated individual. In addition to this we can make observations which are concealed in the one- or two-personal situation, and thus discover *group specific factors* in operation.

As far as the therapist is concerned his most important contribution can be summed up as follows:

(1) He is the representative of the analytic attitude in the group.

(2) He must understand and maintain the group-analytic situation. As a psychoanalyst he is familiar with transference processes. As always the analyst orientates himself on the basis of the total situation in which he works. In the individual situation he will refer part processes to the individual as a whole; in the two-personal situation, to the transference situation; in the group situation, to the group as a whole. He uses this orientation to the total situation as a background for the perspective which he needs; the more so as in his analytic activity, which could in a certain way be said to be a destructive one, he breaks this whole down into parts in order to do justice to them.

What about access to the unconscious? This, as we know, in the two-personal situation in psychoanalysis is based on so-called free association. It has not as yet been well understood that by replacing this 'free association' by 'group association', which the present writer was the first to have done, we make a decisive step regarding method as well as theory. The concept of associations in the individual mind was originally based on the assumption that these were acquired by the individual in his experiences and firmly laid down in his brain. In the two-personal situation this process of giving voice to these 'associations' became already modified by the presence of the second person, the therapist, and his response. In the group, the minds of strangers with a totally different individual conditioning are reacting and responding to each other. If we find – as we do – that their responses, verbal or non-verbal, conscious or unconscious, to each other's productions, can be used as quasi-associations to a common context, we make a totally new assumption. We now treat associations as based on the common ground of unconscious *instinctive understanding* of each other. We no longer take as our basis of operation the conditioning by old experiences based on traces in the brain, on memory traces. Instead we accept that ideas and comments expressed by different members have the value of *unconscious interpretations*. As an observation this had already been understood clearly by Freud and other analysts from the individual situation. Besides it would be quite impossible for obvious reasons, for the group therapist to base his procedure in a group situation on the free association as understood in the individual sense. The relationship which now develops is that of a complex and mutual interaction between members. Only the therapist maintains the analytic attitude and detachment and can see the inner mechanism of this interaction, the unconscious dynamics. It would be quite impossible for him to follow each individual separately at the same time. He focuses on the total interactional field, on the matrix in which these unconscious reactions meet. His background is always, and should consciously be, the group as a whole. Conflicts are now dynamically displayed in the group, and yet they are – as pointed out – not less intrapsychic for that reason.

We cannot go further here into the consequences, for all psychotherapy and theory, of seeing the total situation in the psychotherapeutic small group as one interconnected whole. As group psychotherapists we study human beings and their problems in their full social context, and this study is enriched by opening up otherwise concealed aspects laid bare through pathological conditions which, in studying, we also restore at the same time to normal function.

All psychopathology, psychology, psychotherapy is thus understood to be social, based on intra-psychic processes in their interaction.

Greater freedom, whether looked upon from the group or the individual's point of view, is the result of our successful operations, and the individual gains in independence and strength by his experience of an effective interaction between himself and the group – a two way process operating on many levels. Individuality, which we rightly estimate so highly, emerges in greater spontaneity as the result of group psychotherapy in both patient and therapist alike.

Chapter 2

Significant Features of the Group-Analytic Group in Relation to Other Types of Human Groups

1. GROUPS IN GENERAL

In this chapter we shall pass in review a number of groups as they are found in ordinary life. They will be roughly classified according to certain criteria, derived partly from analytic observation of the dynamics in the therapeutic group. In thus presenting a whole scale of typical groups we hope to bring out more precisely the features of psychiatric therapeutic groups in general, and of group-analytic groups in particular. In any human society we may study there will be an infinite variety of groups, and it is not proposed to describe or classify them fully here.

First of all there are such fundamental social groups as the family, the clan, or even an entire nation. In such groups the members are vitally interdependent; as a class they are best called *communities*. They satisfy basic needs such as food, protection, and sex; human life is never found outside such groups. These fundamental groups, *root groups*, and especially the family group, are in one sense the true objects of treatment, for the mental health of the individual is dependent on his community. However, we are less concerned with the consideration of these root groups in this book, the intention being to study therapeutic groups whose members are initially strangers.

In our culture all sorts of groups arise *spontaneously*, each with a more or less clear purpose. Such groups are not in general organized intentionally, although they may in fact have a high degree of organization and a very definite structure. Thus there are, on the fringe of ordinary social life, groups such as gangs or bands, which have been studied particularly by sociologists and social psychologists. Groups such as neighbourhood groups, children's play groups, and factory groups have also been studied, and innumerable spontaneous groups exist which could be made the object of further study. None of these groups is likely to consult a psychotherapist with a view to treatment, though he may easily find himself up against them in dealing with certain problems, for example delinquency. Their study is therefore of great importance, for it would be impossible to help an individual, say a delinquent boy, without an understanding of his background and its group structure. The study of the dynamics of the special group with which we are concerned, the therapeutic group, throws light in turn on the structure and dynamics of these spontaneous groups in society.

Half of our life is spent in organized bodies or institutions both at work and at leisure, from schools, universities, hospitals, factories, scientific societies to all types of social clubs and associations with special objectives, such as chess clubs, cycling clubs, music circles, in infinite variety. All these societies are indeed important types of groups. They have considerable therapeutic properties, but they are at the same time beset with interpersonal problems. These societies are not as yet – as they should be – made objects of study and treatment as whole groups, but promising beginnings have been made, as in the work of the Tavistock Institute of Human Relations.*

The problems of smaller units, such as for example orchestras, football teams, or troupes of actors, could well be the subject of a more specific group psychotherapeutic approach. This is mentioned here because it can serve as a model for the treatment of a group for the group's sake and with a limited and definite objective in view, such as playing better football.

It is important to keep this type of group in mind as a prototype for any group which is to be treated for its own sake, to improve its mental health, its efficiency, cooperativeness, integration, and so on. It is important because such a group would be the object of treatment for the sake of its functioning as a group. Thus it stands in contradistinction to groups organized for group-analysis, which are, in the last resort, treated not for their own sake but for the sake of the individual members. A 'team' is treated in the first place to improve its efficiency as a team and any benefit that accrues to individual members is a by-product. In a group-analytic group the situation is reversed. The group is treated solely for the benefit of its individual members and its

* See, for example, Elliot Jaques: *The Changing Culture of a Factory*, Tavistock Publications, London, 1951.

efficiency can only be gauged by the extent to which it becomes an efficient instrument for the treatment process.

All these three categories of groups were found within the framework of military psychiatry during the war, especially at the Northfield Neurosis Centre. Inside the Centre all these types of groups were continually forming – spontaneous, underground, undisclosed groups; loosely formed groups with special purposes and functions; and more closely linked and highly organized groups. The special characteristics of each type could be studied. In such a case we can also study the interaction of groups one with another, with their mutual relationships and the influences they exert on each other.

2. OCCUPATION AND THERAPEUTIC ACTIVITY

In order to come closer to a specific delineation of the character of group-analytic groups, it may be useful to establish a few simple terms and some basic considerations.

All the groups we have spoken of so far have tasks, that is, they have definite aims and purposes. This is most important, as we shall presently see, for as a consequence of this fact they generally come together to pursue certain activities. The manifest declared activities of such a group we propose to call the group's 'occupation'. Whereas this manifest occupation has a definite importance, there are usually and perhaps always other occupations going on in the groups, which are not openly declared, which may not be understood by the group and of which it may not even be consciously aware. These 'latent' occupations of the group might well be called its 'preoccupations', and for the understanding of certain occurrences in the group they may be much more relevant than the occupation itself. All groups of this sort have an occupation and some latent preoccupations. The experience we have gained from the analysis of groups shows that this occupation fulfils a very important purpose. It provides the members of the group with a reason for meeting, a means of meeting, and a context for relationships which have a certain impersonal and non-committal quality. Members are able to meet, to share experiences, and to interact emotionally without having to become more involved with one another on a personal level than they wish to be.

A good illustration of the same mechanism is provided by passengers on a ship. They sit together at the bar, or play bridge and deck games. They may come to know each other quite well, exchange jokes, look forward to meeting in the evenings, and, in a sense, become quite intimate, and may yet at the same time communicate to one another almost nothing of their private lives or personal feelings. Generally when the boat reaches its destination they go their separate ways and forget all about each other in a few days.

Analysis of groups shows that group occupations, like the activities of passengers on a boat, serve as a protective screen, a defence against intimate personal interaction. For this very reason psychotherapeutic analytic groups are given *no* occupation, no particular task to perform as a group.

It has been said that these groups occupy themselves with talking. This is correct. Indeed at Northfield we at first called them 'talking groups', in contrast to all other kinds of groups. But they are not talking for talking's sake. As soon as they do this, it becomes clear that they are now talking as if talking *were* their occupation and they are therefore using their conversation as a defence. It is quite a different matter when they talk as a means of communication and not as a defence. In this sense verbal communication is indeed a vital and indispensable part of such a therapeutic group and in a deeper sense an understanding of verbal communication is of special importance for the understanding of the therapeutic process itself.

We have now, perhaps, made clearer some of the important characteristics of group-analytic groups. They are not communities, and their members are not dependent on each other in any way in ordinary life, being in fact total strangers. Nor are they organized societies in the sense in which we have defined this term, nor again are they gangs or bands, or similar in type to any of those groups which form in society at large or within working institutions. They belong by their very nature to the type deliberately brought together for therapeutic purposes. Before we can go further in defining the special features of the group-analytic group, we must therefore consider that whole category of groups which are deliberately organized for therapeutic purposes.

As we turn our attention to such groups, we shall find that

the ordinary life groups just reviewed will help us in our orientation. There is in fact a great variety of 'treatment' groups which we can broadly divide into three categories:

(1) Activity Groups.
(2) Therapeutic Groups.
(3) Psychotherapeutic Groups.

(1) Into the first category fall those groups whose *activities* are deemed to have a therapeutic effect upon their members whether psychological or otherwise. Religious movements like the Oxford Group, various cults, groups promoting physical culture, or recreational or educational activities, discussion groups; all these provide us with examples. A good many of the early therapy groups were basically of this type.

The activities of such groups are organized to further the physical, mental, or spiritual health of the members. Such groups feel their occupations to be of fundamental importance. A physical culture group will feel that physical culture is the essential means for helping its members and all other aspects of its group life will appear secondary. A religious group will feel that its religious convictions and practices are of primary importance and will reject any suggestion that its effect on its members is more related to group dynamics and the personal interaction between them than to these activities. From their point of view, therefore, if these groups are 'therapeutic' they are only accidentally so. They view their function in quite a different light.

(2) To a second category we wish to assign groups which are deliberately arranged for a therapeutic purpose, depending on their character as groups. These groups may be organized round almost any activity – music, drama, puppetry, dancing, art, games, films, discussions, brains trusts, reading classes, and many other activities.

As a result of experience with all of these types of groups and particularly as a result of wartime experience at the Northfield Neurosis Centre, a new idea about group therapy emerged, and came to be increasingly accepted and understood. This idea is that the occupation may be of secondary importance therapeutically, whereas active participation in the group setting may be the essential therapeutic agency. The results of participation will depend on the good or bad effect of the interpersonal relationships which are encountered. The experience at Northfield amply supported this idea and since that time it has been confirmed by parallel experiences and observations from a number of quarters. Thus the effects and dynamics of participation replace the group's occupation as the centre of interest.

It is worth while here to touch on those factors which make for the formation of a 'good group', which further morale and which can foster the health of individuals and even cure their illness. Of paramount importance is the ability of the group's leader to influence its members in a number of ways. He must be able to develop their interest in active and enthusiastic participation in the group's affairs. He must create a spirit of mutual tolerance by bringing into the open many of the frictions which arise so that the group may become aware of the reasons for them. Only thus can the group understand the difficulties within itself and accept responsibility for them. At first everything will depend on good leadership, but good leadership will develop forces in the group which will enable it to take over this function and so free the leader to work at a higher level. It is important that each member, through his group, should have a role to fill in the life of a larger group, and that the larger group should be aware of his place and of its significance. A good group will devise its own modes of meeting, participating, acting, and of discussing and agreeing or disagreeing on its aims.

We must stress that by turning away from the view that a group's 'occupation' is the essence of group activity through which a group must be understood, and by treating the group itself as essential and its occupation as secondary, we take a decisive step. When that step has been taken we propose to speak of group therapy but not yet of group psychotherapy. For group psychotherapy, which is more penetrating, more individualized, more deliberate, and more directed, we need the element of verbal communication.

(3) It is now time for us to define the essential preconditions for *group psychotherapy*, and we shall single out three points:

(*a*) That the group relies on verbal communication.
(*b*) That the individual member is the object of treatment.
(*c*) That the group itself is the main therapeutic agency.

We may say, then, that group psychotherapy uses the group

and its power for therapeutic purposes and is therefore group treatment. But it does not treat the group for the group's sake, to improve its working efficiency, in the way we suggested earlier a team might be treated. The group is treated for the sake of its individual members, and for no other reason. All psychotherapy is, in the last resort, treatment of the individual.

3. GROUP PSYCHOTHERAPY AND ANALYTIC GROUP PSYCHOTHERAPY

It would be true to say that the factors we have enumerated are essential for group psychotherapy. If we now go one step further towards analytic group psychotherapy and in particular towards *group-analytic psychotherapy*, we must make clear the further steps which have to be taken before group psychotherapy can become analytic group psychotherapy.

We shall presently be describing many factors which are necessary to bring about this transformation but the most basic can be outlined here. They are:

(1) That verbal communication is changed into 'group-association'. This implies that discussion in the group shall not be discussion in the ordinary sense of the word but something described as 'free-floating discussion'. It is the group-analytic equivalent of what is known as 'free association' in psychoanalysis.

(2) That the material produced in the group and the actions and interactions of its members are 'analysed'; they are voiced, interpreted, and studied by the group. This means that not only the dynamic processes of the group but also the analysis of those processes form an integral part of the therapeutic operation.

(3) That the subject matter of the discussion is treated not only with regard to its manifest content, but also with regard to its 'unconscious' content, its latent meaning, according to the principles we have learnt from psychoanalysis. Whereas other psychotherapeutic groups work only or mainly with the manifest content of group discussion, group-analytic therapy uses this manifest content to arrive by a process of analysis and interpretation at the latent content, in a way similar to that by which psychoanalysis uses the manifest content of a dream to discover the latent dream thoughts.

The group-analyst's direction of group processes and his own behaviour differ correspondingly.

4. PSYCHOANALYTIC AND GROUP-ANALYTIC PROCESS

From what has been said it will be understood how statements about group behaviour may be made on the basis of group-analytic observations just as observations in other fields, including other types of psychotherapeutic groups, reflect in the group-analytic group. But only from the study of the group-analytic group can we arrive at theoretical formulations which throw light on the unconscious processes operating also in other groups.

In saying this we are not questioning in any way the psychotherapeutic value of participating in other kinds of groups. Human beings, especially in our own type of community, would probably break down much more often than they do but for the direct and indirect support they receive from participating in social groups. The strength and support provided by participation in a group's activities are provided by all these therapeutic groups and by all forms of psychotherapeutic group in the stricter sense of the term. They are undoubtedly provided also by the group-analytic group. But the help which the patient receives from these group-supportive factors is not the essence of psychotherapy in the analytic group. It is not really the essence of any psychotherapy, which aims at a more radical cure.

In view of what has been said we must ask *what* are the specific characteristics of a therapeutic situation that will make the discovery of unknown and unadmitted motives and motivations and their analysis possible. To answer this question we need first of all to go back and remember what we have learned about the psychoanalytic situation.

Psychoanalysis has taught us firstly to take into consideration that part of the psyche which it calls the 'repressed unconscious'. As we know, this repressed unconscious is manifested in the form of symptoms and also in other products of the mind in a disguised and distorted form. Our Bible, when we seek to understand these distortions and to effect their analysis, is Freud's book *The Interpretation of Dreams*. We wish for our present purposes to use an all-embracing name for this whole task, which can be compared to the deciphering of a code. We propose to call this the task of *translation*. We shall return to this topic in the following chapter.

Another aspect of the psychoanalytic process opens up with the discovery and interpretation of resistances and the analysis of what have been called 'defence mechanisms'. We see that these two aims – to make the unconscious conscious, and to analyse the ego's defence mechanisms – require us to become active agents, and to enter as active agents into the dynamic interaction between the ego and the id.

We have now come to a third basic characteristic of the psychoanalytic situation, indicated already by the fact that we have said 'we enter' or 'the analyst enters'. The psychoanalyst participates in this way, in the interpersonal and intra-psychic dynamic process, and thereby becomes a transference figure. The psychoanalytic situation becomes a transference situation. To allow this transference situation to be analysed, to be subjected to analysis, is the quintessence of all psychoanalytic procedure. A particular attitude on the part of the psychoanalyst is required for this, an attitude of acceptance towards any role ascribed to him by the patient.

The precise nature of the psychoanalyst's role is very much under discussion at the present moment. We need not enter into these matters in our present context because they are of importance in the psychoanalytic field rather than in the group-analytic field. But it may be useful to differentiate between two aspects of the analyst's attitude which are not always kept sufficiently distinctly apart. They are his role as an analyst in the psychoanalytic situation and his role, or absence of role, in his capacity as a private, individual, human citizen. In this latter capacity the psychoanalyst still remains as far as possible out of the picture, ideally entirely so. About the first role opinions differ, and certain developments can be discerned in recent years towards the recognition of a more active participation on the part of the psychoanalyst than was originally deemed to be correct. There are doubts as to the optimal degree of the psychoanalyst's emotional participation, and his implicit and explicit activity in the analysis of the transference situation, but there are no doubts as to the fact of this participation which is recognized by all. There is also no question that certain basic attitudes are required of the psychoanalyst if he is to be in a position to play his part, such as a broad and deep tolerance and acceptance of the patient in every respect.

This so-called psychoanalytic situation is the best existing model of what we mean here by a therapeutic situation. It is a situation in which the patient can freely voice his innermost thoughts towards himself, towards any other person, and towards the analyst. He can be confident that he is not being judged, and that he is fully accepted, whatever he may be or whatever he may disclose. There is in addition the interpretation of the patient's contribution and its communication in meaningful language which he and the analyst can share. Further, by the particular attitude and role which the psychoanalyst takes up, the analysis of the all-important transference situation is made possible.

Let us look at the technical tools which are used to achieve this end. With respect to the translation of the repressed unconscious, the basic tool is free association; that is, the communication of everything in the patient's mind without censorship, in so far as that is possible. The main activity of the analyst is interpretation, especially of the patient's defences. With respect to participation in interpersonal and intra-psychical processes, there is the analyst's particular attitude which characterizes this specific therapeutic situation. With respect to the analysis of transferences, there is the couch on which the patient lies. This guarantees the relative impersonality of the analyst and makes it easier for the patient to project all his phantasies on to him without having to deal with the complicating factor of finding socially suitable forms of expression. The patient feels less need to control facial expression, emotional expression, surprise, laughter, amusement, or shock.

Again, in connexion with the analysis of the transference situation we must notice that the analyst focuses his attention and his interpretation on the relationship between the immediately present situation – the here-and-now – and the patient's past. By doing so he is able to investigate the genetic causes of the patient's illness.

We have gone into a description of the psychoanalytic situation and procedure at some length, partly because we shall have reason to refer to it quite often in the course of this book but mainly because it serves as a model for our present purpose, namely that of defining the place of the group-analytic group inside the spectrum of psychotherapeutic groups in general. Group-analytic procedure relates to other forms of group psychotherapy as the psychoanalytic procedure relates to other forms of individual psychotherapy. The typical features of the individual therapeutic situation have their equivalents in the group, but they are correspondingly changed and transformed.

In the following chapter we shall describe the features of the group-analytic situation which correspond to the psychoanalytic situation. We shall see to what extent and in what ways the essential requirements of psychotherapy are met with in the group. We shall notice the ways in which the two situations correspond and ways in which they differ. Here we have illustrated, on the model of the psychoanalytic situation, the character of a psychotherapeutic situation and more specifically, of an analytic psychotherapeutic situation.

As to the frequent comparison of psychotherapies, whether group or individual, in terms of 'deep' and 'superficial', we do not think that psychotherapeutic approaches can simply be described as differing with respect to their depth. It would seem more useful to replace such terms and to speak, for instance, of 'central' or 'essential' therapy versus 'peripheral' or 'symptomatic' therapy. We could then say of any psychotherapy, whether in groups or in the individual situation, whether short or long, psychoanalytic or not, that it was symptomatic and peripheral psychotherapy or, on the other hand, essential and central. Using the terms as we have defined them, we can say at this point that both psychoanalytic and group-analytic psychotherapy are intended to be basic, radical, central therapies, but that the areas in which they each make their main attack differ. Group-analytic psychotherapy emphasizes the immediate present in the therapeutic transactions (the 'here-and-now') and has a more direct effect on the patient's current life-situation and his behaviour. It reveals less of the patient's individual genetic development and of the origins of his disturbance.

Correspondingly the group-analytic situation cannot be used to anything like the same degree for the analysis of the transference reaction of the individual patient and cannot therefore follow in such detail the individual's unconscious conflicts or the intra-psychic dynamics of his personality. Where this is necessary, or specially desirable, psychoanalytic therapy is indicated. On the other hand the group situation affords a much broader and richer insight into the patient's various modes of action and reaction to different people in different and unforeseen situations under conditions much closer to those of ordinary life. The patient's transferences will also be clearly manifested; more will be said about this later. There is, however, one additional advantage of the group situation to which attention may be called here. This is the opportunity it affords for the exploration of what may be called the 'social unconscious'. Each individual's feelings and reactions will reflect the influences exerted on him by other individuals in the group and by the group as a whole, however little he is aware of this. The small therapeutic group also represents for its members other people in general, or even the whole community. In this setting the 'social unconscious' is particularly open to exact investigation with results which can be surprising.

The psychoanalytic process might be called a *vertical* analysis. It goes from the surface to the depth, from the present to the past, thinking in terms of hierarchical layers and levels inside the patient's mind. By contrast, group-analysis might be termed a *horizontal* analysis, in terms of its special features just indicated.

In the next chapter we shall be discussing those features of the group-analytic situation which make it a therapeutic one in the full meaning of the term. But before we do this we still have to notice a view of neurosis which differs from the usual one in its stress on the suprapersonal element. In this view the emphasis is placed on the nuclear and essential significance of disturbed interpersonal relationships for the genesis, understanding, and treatment of neurosis. This view applies equally to psychopathic and deviant behaviour (delinquency, perversion), in a varying degree to psychoses and even physical diseases, and, of course, to such manifestations of inner conflict as accident proneness, inefficiency, disharmony, bad luck, and the like.

Chapter 3

Patients and their Background, and the Group-Analytic Process

1. PATIENTS AND THEIR COMPLAINTS

Our patients come from all walks of life. They are of all ages and as often men as women. Clinically, they are mostly so-called psycho-neurotics. Others would be labelled psychotic, depressed, psychopathic, psychosomatic, or suffering from particular aberrations in their sexual life. We have however learned that these labels have a limited value only, and that people who can be cured or considerably improved may belóng to any of these categories.

It is on the whole true to say that all patients suitable for psychotherapeutic treatment individually should also be suitable for group treatment. However, patients whose problems mainly and manifestly concern a very intimate aspect of their lives, e.g. overt sexual disturbances such as frigidity in women or impotence in men, or homosexuality, are. as a rule better suited in a group which is particularly selected and arranged for them, or for individual treatment.

Undoubtedly, for some conditions and some personalities the individual situation is preferable. What is less well understood and perhaps more surprising: there are many patients for whom the group situation is definitely to be preferred. In the course of this book we shall have occasion to say something more about the reasons for this, and about selection. The finer points of selection and diagnosis, the arrangements, the matching up of suitable groups, are not so much matters for us here as technical problems for the expert. But we shall in the following pages say something of the sort of problems those patients present whom we can encourage to join a therapeutic group.

The nature of the patients' complaints vary enormously, yet they show repetitive patterns which are characteristic and typical of special conditions and particular problems. Usually patients come with a mixture of somatic and psychological complaints. For instance, people may complain of dizzy spells or of fainting attacks, of headaches, digestive disturbances, pains in the heart, colics, and so on. Generally they have had a medical examination, and have often been to several doctors and specialists, and sometimes have even had lengthy treatment. In many cases these doctors have told the patients that there was nothing wrong with them, and that they were simply suffering from 'nerves'.

In some cases we get the impression that the practitioner eventually got tired of them, or impatient, or even annoyed, quite understandably in view of his 'medical' training and orientation, and therefore sent them to us. But today an increasing number of practitioners send such patients from a real understanding of the nature of psychological illness. They have themselves been able to elicit certain pathogenic factors in the patient's life, and have a good idea of the type of problem which is troubling the patient.

Another type of patient does not come through a doctor at all, but has heard through friends, through reading, or through films, plays, or radio talks about psychological treatment and has come more or less on his own initiative.

We must make another very important distinction here between patients. There is the patient who comes to us at his own request, or because he himself feels in need of treatment, and there is the patient who does not really come on his own initiative at all, but because somebody else, the wife or husband, father or mother has urged him to come. Or the second type of patient may come because he has got into some sort of trouble at his office, or even with the law, and this provides the immediate reason for seeking our assistance. This distinction is important when we come to judge his condition and the outlook for treatment.

Now assuming, as we have so far, that the patient's complaints are mainly somatic, the patient when he is told that there is nothing the matter with him may frankly express his disbelief and dis satisfaction. The patient, consciously or not, far under the surface, remains convinced that he is ill, and believes that the doctor has not yet found the cause but that it will eventually emerge. This attitude can vary greatly in strength and depth. These patients often respond very well when the deeper sources of their fear and anxiety are understood and can be convincingly approached by the doctor. On the other hand some patients will superficially accept the doctor's verdict, but will remain convinced unconsciously of their illness and will resist all attempts to uncover their underlying mental anxiety. They may eventually yield to prolonged and exhaustive treatment. One of the reasons for this second reaction is that the conviction of being ill, usually severely ill, is based on deep and pernicious feelings of guilt which are unconscious. In such cases, paradoxical as it may seem, the patient would be really relieved if his dreaded illness were in actual fact discovered. Disturbances of this kind vary widely in complexity and depth and, as we have said before, their treatment is a matter for the expert. They can often be cured for all practical purposes although at first the patient may resolutely resist any attempt to connect his illness with his psychological problems.

Yet another type are not fundamentally in need of the conviction that they are really and seriously ill. But at the same time they do not understand how a headache, or a paralysis of the arm, or an incapacity to swallow or sleep, can be connected with a psychological problem. While they may be quite ready to answer questions, it is not difficult to discover in their attitude a certain feeling of satisfaction with their condition. They are not easily to be shaken out of this feeling, and they fall back, again and again, on hopes that the physician will be able to give them something which will take their suffering away. This type has always a sort of vested interest in maintaining its symptoms. Their suffering is in truth the outcome of an unbearable mental conflict which they have provisionally resolved by forming a symptom. They have therefore no particular interest in elucidating the painful problems which underlie their symptoms and only want to have the unpleasant part of them taken away or else be told over and over again that nothing can be done and that their condition must be accepted.

2. NEUROSIS AND EQUILIBRIUM

We come here to some of the fundamental facts about mental illness: firstly, that underlying neurotic suffering is always mental conflict, and secondly, that none of these neurotic conditions can be changed onesidedly – can be changed because we decide to change them. Change can only come about when there is a disequilibrium in the personality, an unbalance which demands change and can bring about that change. The therapist works with the forces engendered by this disequilibrium, his task is to direct them towards a new balance in the personality which will be more stable because it does fuller justice to inner needs and the demands of outer reality. For this reason, if a patient has achieved a state of equilibrium, if only by means of his symptoms, as may be the case for example with conversion hysterics, there is little the therapist can do.

Every individual necessarily strives to create a dynamic equilibrium for himself in the world in which he has to live. Therefore, in a sense, every individual at any given moment has established the best equilibrium that he is capable of achieving however precarious it may be. The validity of any individual's solution to the problems which beset him can only be seen and appreciated if we take into account the total life situation in which it has been established. We have to take into account not only the patient standing alone before us but his environment, the things he has to do, the place in which he lives, and the people who surround him.

We can illustrate the point with an example. Let us consider a patient who comes to us with a fear of blushing, or better still, to keep within the field of conversion symptoms, a woman who constantly feels sick when going out in company. This symptom may form a necessary part of the best equilibrium she can achieve. In the consulting-room we may find her relatively at ease, and there seems no sufficient reason for her to give up her sickness. But when we examine her life at home we may find that she has difficulties with her husband, that they have scenes in which she punishes him and he attacks her, and the security of her married life is threatened. Or we may find that she is a single woman who has to work for a living, or face severe consequences, who finds her situation at the office or her daily journey there intolerable and, thus, her equilibrium threatened.

A physical illness is understood and recognized, everybody can see it. The patient will get sympathy, special diets, medicine, and holidays. Whereas in the case of nervous trouble, we find as a rule, that neither the patient's doctor, nor his family, nor his friends and workmates, show any sympathy but rather an almost open disapproval. He will usually be advised to pull himself together, to exert some will-power, or to forget about it.

It is fairly easy to see why the majority of people in the patient's environment take up this attitude. Neurosis is in fact an extremely widespread condition, and even those who are rightly considered normal and healthy very often have some weak spots themselves. They have to guard and defend themselves against these in order to maintain their own integrity. In doing so they use just those means of defence, such as 'pulling themselves together', which they recommend to the neurotic sufferer. For this reason anyone like the patient who fails to maintain his control is a threat to their own precarious balance. He appears to them as a dangerous traitor who 'lets the side down'. This hostile reaction to neurotic illness is a commonly observable fact of everyday life. It repeats itself in the therapeutic group and can there be dealt with to the great benefit of all concerned, and can also be studied in its finer and more subtle implications.

In practice most patients come to us with a mixture of physical and psychological symptoms. A patient will say, perhaps, that he suffers from indigestion, constipation, and occasional headaches. He will then also report that he feels anxious in a crowd, or that he has frightening ideas that some catastrophe will happen to somebody dear to him, or that he occasionally wakes up with a nightmare. He will usually agree that his mind is not at ease, but will very often prefer to see no connexion between this and his physical ailments.

3. PSYCHOLOGICAL SYMPTOMS AND TRANSLATION

Let us now turn to a category of people who, at first sight, seem easier to approach – those who suffer from frankly psychological symptoms, symptoms of a mental character. In these cases, too, the symptoms are legion. They may consist of embarrassments, anxieties, fears, compulsions, sleeplessness, or irrational worries. Or again they may be phobic: the patients who cannot cross streets or cannot tolerate being in an enclosed place, or cannot travel in a train, or fear that they will suddenly drop down dead. Some patients are subject to unreasonable impulses sometimes of a most terrifying kind: for example that they will injure their children or wives. Some cannot concentrate, or cannot write, or cannot pass examinations, or they feel direct fear in connexion with sexual relationships. Others may have observed that they always get into trouble in particular circumstances, or that they cannot stand up for themselves, or cannot get promotion when they should, or have severe panic attacks. There are patients who complain of blushing or fear of blushing, of crippling shyness, of various social inhibitions, of morbid phantasy which they know to be groundless, of feeling despised, or that people secretly laugh at them, watch them, talk about them, or disparage them.

All these symptoms are, at least, clearly psychological and consequently the psychiatrist will find it easier initially to approach this type of patient. Such people very much desire an opportunity to talk about their symptoms, find relief in doing so, and want the psychiatrist to reassure them that they are not going mad – that they can be helped and are going to recover. But it is very rare to meet an individual who feels that the worries which really underlie his complaint are hidden from his knowledge and probably remote from those that apparently drive him to seek help. In other words this type of patient, notwithstanding the psychological character of his complaint, is not necessarily a better subject for psychotherapy than the type with physical symptoms. Both are equally on the defence and both, in a sense, would prefer to be ill rather than know the true nature of their problem which is likely in any case to be mainly below the level of consciousness.

For this reason, part of our work with patients of either of these types, and with many others, is in the nature of a 'translation'. It was Freud who showed us not only that distortion does take place, but how and why it does so and also the methods by which we may hope – in collaboration with the patient – to retranslate these distortions back into original meaning. As is well known, Freud did this in connexion with dreams, and in his classic work *The Interpretation of Dreams* (1900) gave us the basic knowledge and technique which we use in this task.

Just because our patients are so unaware of the meaning of their symptoms, they have a long way to go from the state in which we find them to an elucidation of their problems. Indeed even to awake in them a realization that what they suffer from is due to unresolved mental conflict, a conflict in their own minds, is quite a big step. It is in fact very rare for these patients to come and complain of problems, but if they do they will almost certainly complain about the 'wrong' ones.

4. PSYCHOLOGICAL AND PHYSICAL ILLNESS

What we have said so far has perhaps given us an idea of the sort of difficulties with which we have to grapple. These difficulties are encountered in treating any problem which psychiatrists call psychogenetic, that is originating in the mind, and are not peculiar to group psychotherapy. We have been dealing in the foregoing pages with psychological illnesses and psychosomatic illnesses, by which we mean physical illnesses whose origins lie wholly or partly in a state of mental conflict.

We must begin by emphasizing that when we call a condition psychological we do not imply that it is either more real or less real than a physical one. Nor do we maintain that there is anything which we meet and deal with in human life which has not got its physical, material side – even in the case of phenomena which are called by such high-sounding names as 'spiritual'. On the contrary, we believe that everything which happens in the human organism can be looked upon from both aspects: the physiological as well as the psychological or mental. We may fairly ask in the face of any given illness where is the best point to apply a therapeutic lever, and in this respect imagine the various processes on a scale, ranging from the physical at one end to the psychological at the other. This is a practical problem and we may have to apply our therapy simultaneously at several points, but usually we find there is one optimal point.

In a similar way we can also ask where on this same scale the illness or disturbance lies. Ideally and theoretically treatment should correspond in kind to the nature of the illness: physical illness to be treated by physical means, psychological disturbance by psychotherapy. In the foregoing we have indicated why this is often not so in practice. Let us once more illustrate the point.

A patient may be infected by certain bacilli as a consequence of which his heart has, perhaps, been affected. It is now already too late to combat the infection as such (this may in any case have been mastered by the organism), and all we can now do is to treat and support the heart-muscle or the circulation. By now the best treatment may be entirely psychological in an endeavour to bring about greater peace of mind, better capacity for enjoyment and relaxation, and so forth. Or to take a crude example from the field of nervous illness, a patient may have had an accident which we can see on closer examination was in fact an unconscious attempt at suicide. However, at the moment he has a broken leg and concussion of the brain. Obviously we must first treat the fracture and concussion, which will demand the application of surgical techniques, and only later shall we be able to approach the depressive factors in the patient's personality which caused him to involve himself in a serious accident. Conversely we sometimes come across illnesses which start as a *bona fide* physical disease but continue as a complaint which best lends itself to a psychological approach.

5. THE BASIS OF PSYCHOANALYSIS AND GROUP-ANALYSIS

Such differentiations as we have just been making can only be made on a psychological level of thought. The psychological level is the highest because it is the only one which can take into account the patient's whole personality and circumstances. On this level we can determine even early stages of organic disturbance, and sometimes can determine them earlier and with greater precision than by physical means. On this level we can also assess how far the processes of an illness can be reversed by psychological means.

Unconscious conflict in early childhood development is always at the root of psychogenetic disturbances and manifests itself in the patient's reaction to the therapist in the so-called transference situation, where past and present meet. In individual treatment we rely mainly on the transference relationship between therapist and patient to bring about necessary changes. It also manifests itself within his total field of interaction with others. For the study of this wider field and of the location and constellation of his disturbance within its complex network of human relationships the group situation provides an indispensable means of bringing essential patterns into focus. Within the group-analytic situation we have, instead of the individual transference relationship between patient and therapist, a whole spectrum of relationships in active operation before our eyes.

When we come to study the individual origins of a psychogenetic disturbance we are drawn far back into the patient's past; and so it may be worth while to recapitulate once more the characteristics of this relationship between past and present. Psychoanalysis is occupied at one and the same time with the task of what we have called 'translation' – that is, the translation and interpretation of the raw material presented by the patient in the form of free association – and with the relationship which develops in analysis between therapist and patient. This relationship is called a 'transference relationship' because it contains in essence the relationship which the patient formed in early childhood with the most important persons in his environment (usually the parents or their substitutes). These relationships persist below consciousness in the patient's mind and continue to construct the pattern of his relationships to other people in adult life. They are unconscious partly because they have never been conscious, in the sense of accessible to memory, partly because they include deeply repressed feelings of desire, hope, and fear towards the parents, and partly because they have become established by a complicated process of internalization, at the very core of the patient's ego and super-ego. These deep, inner, relationships established in early childhood, become alive again in the so-called transference relationship. Psychoanalysis has shown both that neurotic people suffer from unconscious conflict, and that this conflict is, at its core, a conflict with internalized parental figures.

The phenomena of neurotic illness, which psychoanalysis has studied in the individual therapeutic situation, must of course also appear in the group situation. We shall therefore have to show how they appear in the group and to note similarities and differences between the operation of individual analysis and group-analysis (see Table overleaf).

We shall be dealing with these questions throughout this book but we can note at once certain essential points. The group situation also revives and brings to light the deep and central forces underlying mental conflict. They appear in the way in which members of a group-analytic group relate to the conductor on the one hand and to their fellow patients individually and as a group on the other. But the transference situation in the group is on a much broader front. The individual patient's transference relationship to the conductor or to any other member of the group cannot develop to anything like the same extent as in psychoanalysis and be analysed *vertically* (as we call it) to anything like the same degree. Instead, transference in depth and in its regressive

	Psychoanalysis	*Group-analysis*
Raw material as to subject matter	**Verbal communication, relaxed control**	
	'Free association' of patient	**Spontaneous contributions of members 'Free floating discussion' 'Free group association'**
Translation	**Making repressed unconscious conscious**	
From symptom to meaning From complaint to problem (conflict)	**Interpretation by psychoanalyst**	**Interpretation by group-analyst with the active participation of all members Group-as-a-whole as background of interpretation**
Resistances, defences	**Made conscious**	**Made conscious, including collective and interactional modes**
	Behaviour and expressive (non-verbal) communication	
Raw material as to relationship	**Two-personal situation**	**Multipersonal situation**
	Transference, regressive, infantile	**Multiple transference relationships**
	Counter transference	
	Relations to other people are *outside* the T-situation	***Within* T-situation**
Nature of therapeutic (transference) relationship	**Regression encouraged by situation**	**Regression not encouraged by situation**
	Relative anonymity and passivity of psychoanalyst	**Relatively realistic role by group-analyst and interaction with others**
	Transference neurosis fully established	**Transference neurosis not fully established**
	Problem of dependence and fixation on psychoanalyst	**Less dependency problem**
	No manipulation of transference situation	
Therapeutic processes and principles	**Emphasis on insight and on contrast between past and present**	**In addition: emphasis on reaction and experience in the present situation ('here-and-now') Corrective experience 'Ego-training in action'**

character is more in the background, and the *horizontal*, contemporary plane presents itself for relational operations.

This fact has certain consequences and imposes certain limitations on the value of group treatment in cases which require a complete, detailed, and systematic revision of childhood experiences and childhood neurosis. There are a number of people for whom this is not absolutely necessary even though it might be desirable. These often show that when the greatly amplified and intensified horizontal analysis is taken into consideration, enough vertical analysis of their problems can be done in a group to enable them to make decisive personal readjustment. We shall return to this point when we come to speak of the practical application of group-analysis where such considerations are of particular importance.

Our conclusion at this stage is then, that while some conditions are more suitable for psychoanalytic treatment, other very important ones yield more readily to the horizontal group approach, and for the moment we shall leave the matter there.

6. THE HUMAN ENVIRONMENT

We come now to another point in connexion with that transference relationship which stands particularly and specifically in the foreground of psychoanalytic treatment. However great the importance of transference in all human relationships – and therefore also in our groups – it is equally important to observe and to operate with other relationships which belong to the existing life situation of the patient and which manifest themselves much more fully in the therapeutic group. It is only by observing both the transference characteristics and the reality characteristics of a relationship and by noting how they contrast, overlap, and interact that we can do full justice to the facts before us.

What we wish to underline is that all the disturbances we have touched on so far are essentially and integrally bound up with human relationships. Our experience with groups and especially with analytic groups in recent years has brought this out much more clearly than ever before. These disturbances affect first the patient's relationships with those nearest to him, and any dislocation in these relationships is the first indication we get of mental illness, be it light or severe. Furthermore, the best approach to the treatment of these disturbances lies through the analysis, correction, and deeper understanding of human relationships. Herein lies the essence of therapy and it is best applied in a human group – a group of a particular kind.

We can go still further and say that in our observation none of the disturbances we have mentioned is really confined to the person who comes to us as a patient. They are not simply a function of his individual personality, not even in their symptomatic aspect, but are functions of a whole nexus of relationships between many people. For example, a marital disturbance is always a matter between at least two people and, as soon as we study the conflict between this couple, we find it involves other people, perhaps a mother-in-law towards whom each partner feels differently, and this in turn involves each partner's earlier relationships to his or her parents and brothers and sisters. Again we may find that the irritating mother-in-law only reacts to the original couple in the way she does because her own father, brother, or son is involved, and so the expanding network of implicated relationship grows. Even to describe adequately and accurately the simplest case, we could almost say even to describe a single symptom, we have to refer to an interacting network of human relationships from which it grows.

All this leads us to the general formulation that the disturbance which we see in front of us, embodied in a particular patient, is in fact the expression of a disturbed balance in a total field of interaction which involves a number of different people as participants. The patient who comes to us is more or less unaware of all this and, being a wholehearted participant who plays his full part in this network of forces, he wants to be helped without being forced to cooperate in any really basic changes. That is, he wants to leave the situation as a whole just as it is, but to be enabled to do so without paying the price for this in terms of illness, without cost to himself. He may even want our help to do harm or to put someone else within his field of relationships in the wrong. It is rare that a patient comes with the wish to take responsibility for his problems, or to be put in a position to tackle his problems himself and settle outstanding issues. Usually he comes with the unconscious wish to change his conflict into some form of suffering or symptom, for which he can pretend to want treatment, and in this way lay the onus of his problems on his doctor. In the face of this situation, we, unlike the patient, know that a real change is needed. Where the patient really wants to make no fundamental change we want to achieve a fundamental change in him and, as a necessary result, in the relations between him and the other people involved. We can now see better perhaps that there are, apart from the defensive forces in the person himself, also defences opposing changes in the total field.

These often come out quite dramatically in the course of treatment, when the other people involved in the patient's illness and who in a way drive him to seek help, begin to react, unconsciously and indirectly but very obviously, against any change in the patient. This reaction is generally expressed as opposition to a development which would make the patient less dependent on them and more able to stand up for himself and against their claims on him. These interactions between the patient and his human environment are strongly and deeply felt. We are watching here the play of passionate emotional feelings and we conclude from this that the changes we have initiated are taking place on fundamental levels of the patient's personality. This should not really surprise us, if we remember that neurotic suffering of any kind is the result of conflict – conflict between interacting personalities and within the interacting personalities – and represents a tentative solution of that conflict, a compromise which involves much suffering but at the same time much satisfaction and the avoidance of something judged more formidable than the suffering. It is therefore inevitable that any treatment which touches the deeper conflict and seeks a new resolution of it will also entail suffering.

7. THE CONSTRUCTION OF THE GROUP SITUATION

After this brief survey of the field, we can now proceed to develop our ideas, firstly on how to construct a situation in which the many considerations we have raised can be met, and secondly on how that therapy can be adapted to the needs of the patients.

The situation which we want must make it possible to achieve the following:

(*a*) What we have called *translation*. For this we need the communication of material that would normally be censored, so that we can arrive, with the help of this material by steps and stages, at the repressed and unconscious meaning of the patient's communications. We want means of communication under reduced censorship.

(*b*) This reduced censorship must apply also to the patient's relationship to others, including the conductor. This very important feature enables us to approach what might be called the social unconscious, i.e. such social relationships as are not usually revealed, or are not even conscious.

(*c*) That the personalities of the group members come to the fore, and become fully and actively engaged. We want members to be completely and vitally interested participants in a situation which concerns them, and to speak and behave as spontaneously as possible.

We realize that these three points are closely interlinked.

What are the main tools with which we achieve these things?

(1) We encourage the relaxation of censorship. We do this by letting the patient–members understand that they are not only permitted, but expected to say anything they think of, anything which comes to mind. We tell them not to allow any of the usual inhibitory considerations to stand in the way of voicing the ideas which come to them spontaneously, whether in relation to something someone else has brought up or not brought up, or in relation to the other members of this particular group.

We have described the type of conversation which gradually develops under these conditions as 'free-floating discussion', because this is the form it very often takes, but we might also call it 'free group association'. What we mean by this is simply that we do not give the group any theme, programme, or points for discussion, nor do we ask for anyone's opinion, as one would for instance in a committee. Instead we leave discussion entirely to the spontaneous mood of the group and its members, fully accepting whatever comes up at each moment of each session. We admit any communication, whether or not it seems to have a connexion with what has been going on before.

We use this material for translation and interpretation, but instead of this being mainly the task of the therapist we further and stimulate the active participation of the whole group.

As a result the responses to any communication increasingly tend to assume one of three forms. Either – in classic style – they are associations, ideas which come to members' minds, whether they seem to have a bearing or not. Or they may be interpretations, members offering suggestions as to the real meaning of the communications. Or, finally, they may be reactions against the communications; that is defensive responses.

In addition we look for the response of the group as a whole to the communications of the individual patient, just as we view the individual patient's communication as coming from the group, through the mouthpiece of the speaker.

(2) With regard to the frank disclosure of personal feelings and experience, and of feelings toward other members of the group, this point is mainly achieved by the conductor's attitude. The conductor accepts and even encourages such statements as might not be made in an ordinary social situation, and which are free or relatively free of censorship. The total atmosphere – the group-analytic atmosphere – as set by the conductor, is one of tolerance and encouragement for such free disclosures. This is the salient point here.

Very soon, of course, the members of the group will understand the mutual nature of exchanges. They will see that just as they can tell someone else what they think or feel about him (or her), they must also tolerate being told the same sort of things. They very soon discover the mutual benefit of such communications. They come to realize that the person who makes an observation, speaks as much about himself as about the other person, and that by pointing out something, whether correctly or incorrectly, to another person, he helps the latter's self-knowledge. All this is quite apart from the additional comments and judgements which are contributed by the rest of the group and by the conductor.

This second point is a particularly good illustration of how the group uses its own resources. It is an activity which is only possible in a group-setting, with its multitude of interrelationships.

(3) From what has just been said about the activities of the group, it can be seen that the members of such a group are active participants. They are engaged actively in the therapeutic process, and are not merely 'recipients' of treatment as they so very much wish to be.

They are in the thick of things, and are confronted continuously with situations which they have to meet actively. They are, therefore, in a sense, undergoing a training in interpersonal relationships, but undergoing it in a protected sphere, in that the situation is not part of ordinary life. Events in the group are taken up in a different way and with different consequences from events in life outside.

We can see now why it is important for the group to have no occupation, and no reason for existing beyond itself, no task to perform at its meetings.

It is this absence of any programme which automatically brings the personalities of members to the fore in the way we have described. They are confronted with the ever-changing task of adjusting personal relationships which continuously develop in unusual and unexpected ways. The protective screen of an occupation behind which they can hide in any other form of social group is taken away. By removing this screen and by throwing the group back on free-floating discussion, we create a situation which can meet the demands of therapy outlined earlier in this chapter.

It must be understood that neither in the individual situation nor in the group situation is the cooperation of either patient or therapist perfect. It is not always within a person's power to overcome the censorship in his own mind. However, the very fact that the patients come to us because they are suffering and in need of help acts as a driving force towards cooperation in the therapeutic situation.

The impetus to self-revelation in a group provided by the patient's suffering is of enormous value from the point of view of scientific research. It enables us to study interactions which in other circumstances would be hidden, and to check many of our findings with the persons concerned.

We may perhaps be asked why participation in such a group should be therapeutic, and we shall answer this question more extensively in Chapter 7. But we can already, from what we have said, enumerate certain factors. Firstly, there is the supportive effect that participation in any moderately well-meaning group has. Secondly, there are the analytic factors which interest us more particularly. The group-analytic situation brings to light unconscious meaning, unconscious motivation, and interpersonal reactions which are unknown, unconscious though in a different sense. During this work of discovery the patient experiences, and understands in a way that touches deep emotional feelings and not merely his intellect, his own reactions to others, his mistakes, and his misjudgements. Through comparison of his own estimate of the nature and cause of disturbance in himself and others with those of his fellow members, he learns to modify them. The group-analytic process releases a host of factors which operate to increase the patient's insight and forms a sort of training ground where his relationships with other people can be tested.

Thirdly, we must point to the therapeutic effect of the very steps the group as a whole, and each individual member of it, has to take in order to make himself understood and to feel that he understands others. The mental work and the interpersonal effort needed to secure ever-improving communication is of central importance for the therapeutic process and we shall enlarge on this in the theoretical part of this book.

It has been shown by some people who have had experience of groups in industry, where problems between the staff and the management, including personal problems, have been freely faced, and where certain characteristics of the therapeutic situation have been duplicated, that similar mechanisms play a part. There is no doubt they do, and this leads us to ask whether there are any specific therapeutic factors peculiar to the group-analytic situation alone.

We do not think that there are any such factors which may not appear in some guise in other types of group. What distinguishes our analytic groups is not the presence of certain unique factors, but the particular combination of the several factors which we have already enumerated, and the way in which they are used.

There is the free-floating verbal communication carried to an extreme point; there is the maximum reduction of censorship with regard to the content of contributions and to the expression of personal and interpersonal feelings; there is the attitude of the conductor, who not only actively cultivates and maintains the group atmosphere and the active participation of members, but also allows himself to become a transference figure in the psychoanalytic sense and accepts the changing roles which the group assign him; there is the emphasis on the unconscious repressed in the psychoanalytic and on the interpersonal and social unconscious in the group-analytic sense; there is analysis and interpretation of the material produced by the group.

Group Psychotherapy

It is the concerted application of all these elements in a judiciously selected interplay which makes a situation therapeutic. The psychoanalytic situation is known in such a capacity as a 'transference situation'. Some writers declare the group therapeutic situation to be not more and not less than a transference situation in a group setting. We propose to signify those properties of a (psycho-) therapeutic situation which make it essentially therapeutic by the symbol 'T'.

In the T-situation past and present must meet. The past – which was unconscious, repressed, or never experienced in such form as could be recalled except through repetition in behaviour – is accepted as present in the T-situation.

In connexion with this, it is one of the relevant conditions that the participants in a group-analytic group are strangers except for their contact within the group. The very personal and real emotions and attitudes between members thus remain inside the T-situation, and are prevented from spilling over into ordinary life. There are, however, in our opinion, other ingredients, equally essential, which make a situation therapeutic. Whereas the T-situation is a transference situation ($T = tr$) it has other features as well, as we have indicated and we can therefore formulate: $T = tr + x$.

Chapter 4

Some Technical and Practical Aspects of the Group-Analytic Situation

1. THERAPY AND RESEARCH

Every therapeutic episode can be regarded somewhat loosely as an experiment or essay in research. This concomitance of treatment and research is now a commonplace in medicine and is largely responsible for advances in the field of therapy. For many psychotherapists, however, even this moderate scientific attitude is felt to interpose an emotional distance between the therapist and his patient. Research is interpreted as an active interference with the spontaneous evolution of the therapeutic relationship.

This shows a misunderstanding of the nature of therapeutic research. Such research is a by-product of the spontaneous therapeutic process. The therapist remains relatively passive and detached. There is no overt difference in his behaviour. He is a *participant observer*. He does, however, observe with an open mind and tries to view his data without a preconceived bias. That is, he is prepared to learn something new from his findings and not only something old. The 'open mind' is the prerequisite for research. In treatment, you find what you set out to find. In therapeutic research you may find nothing significant – but that would still be something.

To carry it out efficiently, certain special arrangements need to be made, so that the observations can be undertaken against a fairly steady background – one that can be approximately reproduced by other workers. This background is, therefore, an important adjunct to group research. It does not pretend to be 'standardized' in the strict sense of the word, but it is reasonably constant and well-defined within certain flexible limits.

The problem has been to design a therapeutic situation to meet the two simultaneous requirements of therapy and research, and keeping in mind the reservations already discussed, the two arrangements dovetail most effectively into each other. To take one example: the psychoanalytic situation meets these twin demands by an arrangement which is generally accepted by psychoanalysts and gives consistency and coherence to their data. The patient lies on a couch and the analyst sits behind and beyond his visual range. The reason for this arrangement is found in the theory underlying the psychoanalytic technique. This lays emphasis on the infantile conflicts which are transferred from the invisible parents in the past to the invisible analyst in the present. Invisibility favours this transference of the inner parental image, and the therapist is free to become a representative in phantasy of either parent, irrespective of his or her sex.

The group situation, on the other hand, belongs much more to 'real' life in the present, the 'here-and-now', and to problems of current adjustment. Full cognizance is taken of the unconscious background to these problems, but the analysis is not primarily directed towards the resolution of the infantile conflicts in transference.

The group-analyst, therefore, has less need to hide himself. He makes himself part of the present problem, and faces the swirl of conflict in the group as a real person in his own right. Like the psychoanalyst, he remains essentially passive and detached; not, however, in order to favour projection but to encourage group interaction. Over-activity on his part may lead to an authoritarian 'fixation' of the group because of their immature needs for a leader. Having created an appropriate and dynamic situation for therapy, the group-analyst, like the psychoanalyst, can let the patient get on with the problem of curing himself with as little interference as possible.

This special situation for group psychotherapy is the result of long and patient inquiry into the therapeutic possibilities of the group. It is an empirical arrangement based on the hard experience of trial and error, and success. Looking at the situation as a whole, it can be described first in terms of the material arrangements and then from the purely psychological angle. The material arrangements have, of course, their important psychological concomitants which will also be mentioned.

2. MATERIAL ARRANGEMENTS

The group room should be quiet, impersonally furnished, and

of sufficient size to contain a small intimate circle of chairs in which the group members can sit comfortably within easy talking and watching distance of each other. It is customary to leave the central space of the circle furnished only with a small table. This leaves nothing to hide behind, so that the members of the circle are exposing those expressive and revealing parts – the face, the hands, and the feet – which 'talk' their 'body language' even during silent periods of the session. The therapist is one of the circle and equally 'vulnerable' to the eye.

What is the possible psychological representation of the circle? It is a figure which has always been credited with magical properties and widely utilized in symbolic and metaphorical language ('magic circle', 'best circles', 'circle of friends', 'wheels within wheels'). It has been taken to signify a static compromise, an equilibrium, of peripheral movement to and away from the centre. In the language of physics, these are the centripetal and centrifugal tendencies; and in the language of the emotions, an ambivalence of positive and negative (attracting and repelling, loving and hating) forces. The circle of chairs may then be said to give concrete expression to the distance at which the members will interact best without becoming too anxious or feeling too remote. In stating this, one might recall Schopenhauer's well-known analogy of human beings to hedgehogs. The neurotic 'hedgehogs' of the group circle must decide how close and how far they can be from each other to avoid feeling both the cold and the pricks. When the psychological 'space' between the members is disturbed in the course of treatment, attempts to shift the chairs back or forward will be observed.

The free choice of seats made by members, in relation to each other and to the conductor, is often extremely significant, making due allowance for accidental factors of late-coming and absence. After an initial period of random selection, the circle may 'harden' into a characteristic pattern, an alteration in which may anticipate dynamic alterations in the interpersonal relations. This pattern of assembly furnishes hints, also, as to the functional roles played by the members of the group at any particular time, detecting the emergence of 'deputy leaders', 'favourites', 'scapegoats', and 'pairings'.

A period of psychological resistance may be equally manifested in the resistance to any change in the shape, size, or general configuration of the circle, and any movement, such as the introduction of new members or the leaving of old members, may provoke resentment against the 'prime mover', the therapist.

Group psychotherapists have always laid great stress on the question of numbers. Numbers help to determine the size of the group circle and the amount of group time each member 'imagines' is portioned to him – this may occasion guilt when he feels that he has monopolized more than his due.

Various numerical experiments have been carried out by therapists and their psychological effect on group procedure assessed. It was necessary to learn from such basic experience at what point of membership a group became a group, and at what further stage it ceased to be a group and became a crowd. The aims of therapy dictate the necessary numbers, and numbers dictate the limits of therapy. The group arrangements by numbers shown schematically make clear the importance of the numerical factor:

Type of Situation	*Numbers*
Self-analysis	1
Psychoanalysis	2
For the group to work at all	3
For the group to be at all representative	5
Optimal range	7–8
'Free' discussion group	10–20
Social club therapy	—
Community therapy	—

From the shape and size we pass next to structure, which we will deal with in some detail, as this is the factor that gives a group its special recognizable character.

In the first place, there is the question of fixity or plasticity of the membership structure. Is the group 'closed' to new members or does it remain 'open'? And if it remains open, are the new members introduced at relatively infrequent intervals (a slow-open group) or fairly frequently (the open group)?

The open group is an important form of the therapeutic group, but not the most essential, useful, or intensive. It has been incorporated into treatment schemes at the Maudsley Out-patient Psychotherapy Department as a preparatory therapeutic experience. Some patients spend their whole treatment time in them, whereas others may move on into individual psychotherapy or into closed groups. Open groups are also suitable for patients who have had intensive therapy of some sort and require some 'after-care' help as a finishing measure. The so-called slow-open group is a compromise formation between the open and the closed, acknowledging that circumstances, particularly in private practice, seldom permit a group to remain closed over any great length of time. Losses may occur and may reduce the group membership to a sub-optimal level, unless replenished periodically. The slow-open group is 'the maid of all work' in group practice and is eminently adaptable to different requirements.

The closed groups provide the best environment for very intensive therapy, especially when the members have been well matched. It is the ideal group for research into individual and group psychopathology, and we shall give some examples in a subsequent chapter of this application. This form of group can also be usefully time-limited.

Selective procedures, carefully carried out, may render the conductor's task a much lighter one.

General principles. Any patient considered likely to benefit from psychotherapy, particularly analytic psychotherapy, would also, in general, be considered suitable for group psychotherapy. For some patients the individual situation may be preferable, for others the group; but in the overlapping area when either would do, such practical considerations as time and money may influence the choice in favour of the group method.

As a rule, in the process of selection, a great deal of common ground is already taken for granted. For example, we know that our patients will be talking the same language against the same background of national feeling and participating in all the imponderables that go to make up a pattern of culture.

To these basic common experiences, we can add other shared conditions, such as age, sex, religion, social background, intelligence, education, profession, marital status.

A group selected on these general factors could not be called a highly selected group, but they are basic to more specific selection. They are so obvious, like the clothes a person habitually wears, that one hardly thinks about them. And yet how significant they are in all their trivial detail in the setting of the group!

Whereas in individual psychotherapy they are usually classed as external, superficial, and unessential, the group reveals them in all their intrinsic importance for treatment. This then is the revolutionary quality of the group as a therapeutic situation, *which is a total situation*, and to which all these factors contribute. A patient might come to an analyst with an obsessional neurosis; it would be of secondary consideration that he happened also to be a Roman Catholic, a man, a doctor, etc.; but these are an essential part of the whole structure of the therapeutic relationship.

Specific principles of selection. The more specific principles can be classified on the basis of the sifting they effect, ranging from coarse to very fine. Three main categories based on clinical assessment or diagnosis emerge:

(1) *The heterogeneous group.* This is a 'mixed bag' of diagnoses and disturbances which are blended together to make a well-balanced and therapeutically effective mixture. The process of *blending* may be based on diagnoses (psychotics with psychoneurotics), temperament (forthcoming with shy patients), verbal participation (talkers with silent patients), and so on. ... The greater the 'span' between the 'polar' types, the higher the therapeutic potential, if the group can stand it.

(2) *The intermediate group.* Here an attempt is made to match 'personalities' together; but it must be remembered that a single character trait, for example, exuberance, may be the social expression of many unrelated conditions – cyclothymia, psychopathy, epilepsy, a defence against passivity, addiction, etc.

(3) *The homogeneous group.* This is perhaps the most promising type of group from the point of view of research. The patients may be selected on the basis of some syndrome, e.g. a common phobia, the fear that they might harm their children, catch venereal disease, develop cancer, etc.; or on the basis of some common problem, e.g. marital or child guidance problems. Again, it must be borne in mind that similar problems may result in quite different symptoms, whilst similar symptoms may have resulted from quite different problems.

The homogeneous group should be run on *closed* lines, the two factors greatly intensifying the group-analytic process. Certain severe personality disorders – e.g. homosexuality, addiction, delinquency – show possibly more therapeutic promise in this type of group than in any other therapeutic situation except a very long and intensive psychoanalysis.

For practical purposes we prefer the heterogeneous, slow-open group. A time-saving and interesting procedure is to allow the group to carry out its own selection, using the group situation as the test. It must be remembered, however, that not only is the particular patient on trial but also the group; and if the group fails to assimilate the patient, the fault may be equally with the group as with the patient. Nor, if the patient fails at one group, can it be assumed that he is unsuitable for group therapy. He may be a great therapeutic success in a different group.

To allow the group to do its own selecting is to pay particular heed to the group's needs as a group. The therapist, too, in his own selective procedure, may choose his patients on the grounds of suitability for a particular group, on the assumption that what is good for the group must be good for the individual, and this frequently turns out to be the case.

One other structural situation may complicate the picture of the group. Some, none, or all the members of the group may be receiving individual psychotherapy as well. Experience has shown that the most effective combination is for individual therapy to be followed by group therapy as a 'rounding-off' process, or for individual therapy to be preceded by group therapy as a preparatory measure. These combinations are to be preferred to the concurrent use of both, which, if done at all, should be done in an open group and with all the members. The important principle is not to isolate any patient by different treatment or bad selection.

A group session once a week works quite satisfactorily. It is too early to say, judging from our own experience, what the special advantages or disadvantages are of more frequent sessions. These extra sessions should intensify matters considerably and perhaps shorten the total duration of treatment, but practical difficulties render such possibilities rare save in in-patient hospital practice, and the hospital in-patient does not always make the most suitable group patient. With the standard frequency working so well, there seems no great necessity to press for more impracticable procedures.*

* Twice-weekly groups have been held more recently and have been found to be well worth while.

From experience again and on purely empirical grounds, we have found that the best workable time is 1½ hours. It should not be shorter than one hour, and to extend it beyond the hour and a half does not add anything to the session. The group only extends the 'warming-up' period in such a case. Having chosen a suitable length of time it is better to stick to it throughout the treatment, although termination of any particular session should not be brought about too abruptly. It is important that both therapist and members should learn to tolerate the tension of suspended business and carry it away for 'working through' during the week.

How long a course of treatment lasts depends on the nature of the group and on the setting. One would tend to treat open and closed groups, and in-patient and out-patient groups differently in this respect. In hospital practice, although matters are changing rapidly, there are not enough groups as yet available in which patients can stay over a long period. In private practice, on the other hand, it is possible now for individuals to participate for a number of years without causing financial hardship to themselves. Intensive treatment will probably take an average of two to three years (a year having roughly 40–45 sessions). Although good results may be seen even in a period of a few months, we have come to consider nine months as a minimal period. Treatment is generally begun as a timeless task. Closed groups can be usefully run with a predestined duration in mind.

The surgeon rightly demands an aseptic field of activity, although he has at his disposal an elaborate choice of antiseptic and antibiotic measures. He has no wish to multiply his difficulties simply in order to overcome them. The group therapist also likes to do his work with the help of a few psycho-prophylactic provisions which help to make the group a better instrument of therapy.

In the group-analytic groups our practice is to discourage all outside contact between members and thus confine their contacts and communications to the actual treatment session. Meeting outside, visiting each other, developing intimate relationships, etc., all help to bring unnecessary difficulties to the course of treatment.

Arriving punctually and attending regularly are important therapeutic pointers; a fact which can be demonstrated to the beginner vividly by reference to a special record attendance sheet* which plots the week-to-week attendances, punctuality, absences, excuses, etc. From such a record, it can be shown graphically that as soon as a certain amount of irregularity sets in, it may take many weeks before the group is again in the same composition, which makes it improper to draw inferences based on the supposition of a constant situation.

These restrictions are not imposed upon the group by the conductor. He should make it clear what the therapeutic argument is for their maintenance, and then leave it to the group to act on their own conclusions. The group will rarely work consciously against the therapeutic stream except for short periods of defiance against the implicit authority of the conductor. They are already on their way to recovery when they freely accept these simple rules as steps on the way to greater emotional freedom within themselves. The Platonic Socrates, in his theory of knowledge, held the view that men did not choose to do wrong things in preference to the right because they were evil-minded, but because they were muddle-headed and ignorant. What man, asked Socrates, given the choice of doing right or wrong, with full understanding of the choice, would prefer to do wrong? The group therapist also acts on this principle of free choice on the basis of full understanding, and assumes that the group, without any pressure from him, will prefer to take the therapeutic road, even though it is a little rougher.

The prospective group patient would be untrue to life if he failed to show certain fears and misgivings based on misconceptions of the group situation.

In his preliminary meeting with the therapist he may ask several anxious questions and bring up some of his fears. He may ask, for instance, about the risk of 'mental contamination' or 'cross infection', of assimilating other people's troubles and problems and so becoming rather worse than better. Such fears are quite unfounded. Things are not put into people's minds magically, which are not already there. In the group situation, patients come together at the crossroads of their several disturbances and do not take them over from each other.

Another fear is that they will be expected to confess, before strangers, all their intimate 'sins', as in a revivalistic meeting. The

* S. H. Foulkes: *Recording Group-Analytic Sessions*, Group-Analytic Society, London, 1953.

answer to this is that the group itself sets the boundaries for its own communications. The group, being part of outside life, brings in the same standards. Being progressively oriented, it talks more in the language of real life, and less in the infantile, regressed language of the patient on the psychotherapeutic couch. It is true that people do talk more freely in therapeutic groups than in social groups. There are barriers and limits, but these are constantly moved further out and may, at times, be removed altogether. There is no orgy of self-revelation.

Still another fear concerns itself with the worry that information given in the group may leak out, and reach back to their reference. From a wide experience we cannot say we have had any difficulties in this respect, and, moreover, with our knowledge of the workings of a therapeutic group, we would not expect to have any in the future. To a great extent the world outside remains anonymous and unnamed, and references are mostly in very general terms – 'my boss', 'my friend', 'the woman in the shop', and so on.

3. PSYCHOLOGICAL ASPECTS

Having discussed the physical structure and arrangements of the group, we shall now examine the psychological aspects of the situation. What we have already said makes it abundantly clear that the therapeutic group has a protean function, the dimensions of which have yet to be fully explored.

The keynote to the group-analytic situation is its flexibility and its spontaneity, and these two, from the very beginning, give it its specific character. The group meets and shapes itself into a circle. And that is all the formality there is. There is no set topic for discussion, no rules of procedure, no programme, no leader. The conductor may make a few opening remarks, but these remarks are not in any sense a formal instruction to the group or a rule of procedure. It is by his handling of the group, and his reactions to their initial communications that he lets them know what is expected of them in the situation. The procedure grows naturally out of the group experience, and is implicit in the group situation. In this unusual 'climate' of the group, in this 'atmosphere' of easy permissiveness, of free-floating discussion, things begin to happen. And they happen without a great deal of effort on anyone's part, as if they were self-generated by the nature of the situation, which, to a great extent, they are.

There is a rise and fall of feeling and talking and laughing against a kaleidoscopic background of interaction. Every now and then an unaccountable silence occurs, anxiety rises, tension overflows into movement, and every member feels the edge of a new and unexplored territory. Then someone bursts in with a 'tea party' topic of escape, and 'saves' the group from its own further therapeutic development – for the time being. Then they are on the move again – until the next pause. And so it goes on. Not in a straight line, but progressively towards greater understanding.

There are two sets of factors at work in the therapeutic process, the supportive and the analytic.

First, the supportive factor. This function of the group-analytic group is one that it shares with all therapeutic groups. Each member has the feeling of being supported, of being accepted, of being able to talk and of being listened to, of sharing with others, of living through similar emotional experiences as others, of being able to cope with loneliness and isolation. It is the factor of 'belongingness', to use Kurt Lewin's term.

Second, the analytic factor. Like psychoanalysis, group-analysis is an uncovering therapy. Defences are analysed, conflicts bared, and insight into apparently irrational modes of behaviour and interaction is achieved. Each patient both experiences and observes the dynamic processes and disturbances that are generated in the group. This so-called corrective emotional experience is the cornerstone of the whole therapeutic structure.

The group-analytic situation has been compared to a projective test, where the material is alive and multidimensional, and into which each patient must actively thrust his whole personality. The more actively he participates in the process the more therapeutic change is there likely to be. From the observer's end, there are ever-changing patterns of relationships, transient configurations, that alter in a bewildering fashion, and patterns of communication that reflect the basic relationships.

The theory of communication arising from our experience in group-analytic groups is discussed in another chapter. Here the changing patterns observed during the evolution of the group will be outlined. People who come into therapeutic groups arrive with a considerable load of group experience in life. Depending on the nature and degree of their neurotic or psychopathic disturbance, limits will have been set to their ability to interrelate and communicate with others. For the social isolates, the marginal members of society, the hopelessly inadequate, such basic social skills may be at their minimum. These individuals may withdraw into their inner world of experience. In the group they meet, perhaps for the first time, people prepared to accept their communications and establish a two-way system of give and

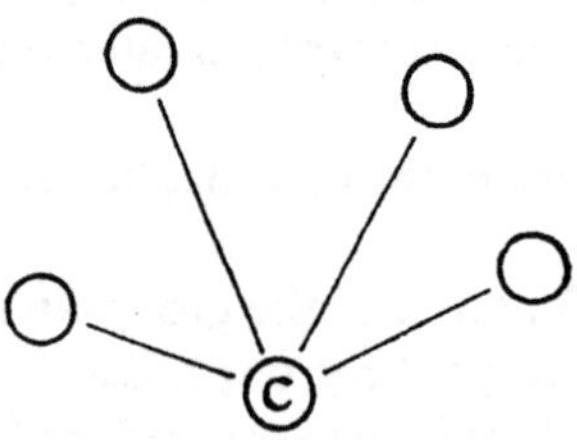

Fig. 1

Leader-centred group with leader-directed communications and simple interrelational patterns

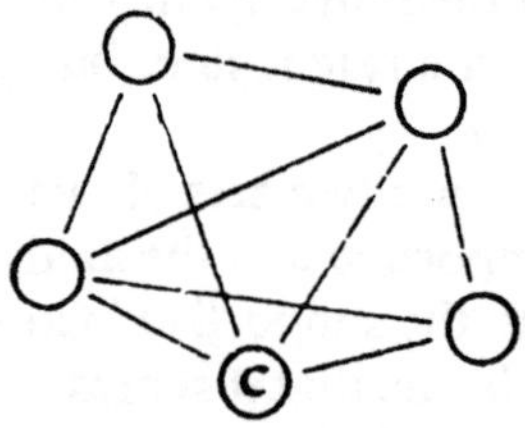

Fig. 2

Group-centred group with group-directed communications and complex interrelational patterns

take. In the early stages the talk of such people will be largely egocentric and self-oriented. A study of serial communications will indicate their inability to interchange ideas. Serial samples may show a patient's strong tendency to soliloquize. In time he may accept ideas from other members but only where they fit in with his own line of thought. Finally genuine interaction may occur and an idea may be assimilated that is foreign to his way of thinking and may break into the egocentric structure of his inner processes. With genuine interaction comes genuine communication which is plastic and modifiable by group experience. He is now ready for a mutative emotional experience that will bring about changes in his social and emotional responses to others, that is, his interpersonal relationships. This is an extreme example of what probably occurs in all groups. Communication follows in the wake of interaction and exhibits comparable changes (Figs. 1 and 2).

This highly schematic representation indicates the dynamic

shifts in interpersonal relationships, verbal interchanges, and leadership attitudes that take place with the setting up of the group-analytic situation.

It will be noticed that the lines of communication tend to shorten with the increasing integration of the group. Discussion is freer and directed towards the open forum. Instead of communicating with each other mainly through the conductor, members are able to communicate directly with each other.

Communication records (a schematic record of all communications made to and from each member) show clearly the relational patterns for any one session (Figs. 3, 4, and 5).

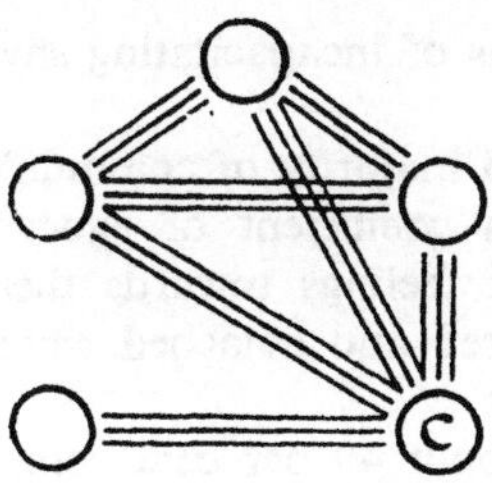

Fig. 3
Isolation

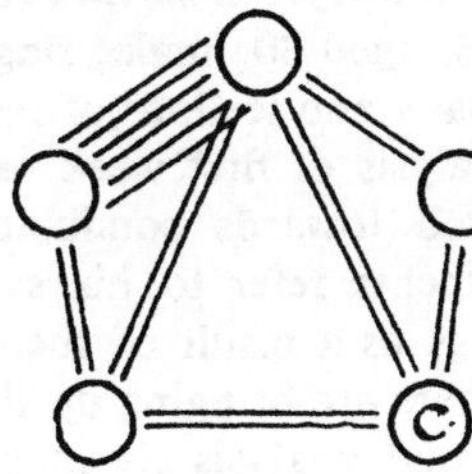

Fig. 4
Sub-grouping

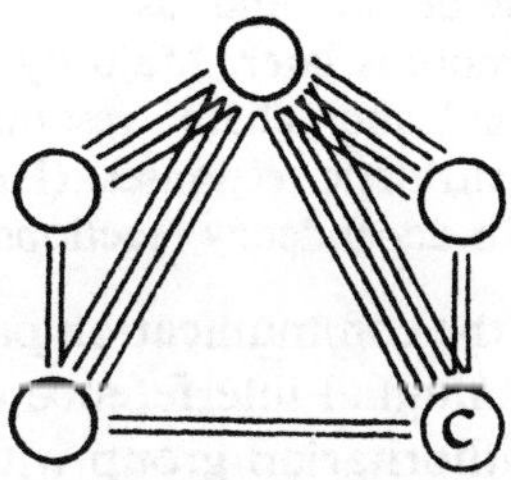

Fig. 5
Monopolism

Communication, here, is taken to mean verbal communication, which is the type of communication most desirable and most encouraged in analytic groups. It increases the 'shareability' of group experiences and brings material more prominently into consciousness. It is, besides, the most effective and most efficient means of communication, and consequently the most effective and most efficient means of therapy.

That the individual's mode of communication changes in the course of group treatment can best be shown by an illustration.

Group Psychotherapy

The socialization effect, the therapeutic effect, and the communication effect run hand in hand, and it is difficult to separate them. The egocentric, narcissistic individual becomes more socially oriented, as his range of sharing and communication grows. A functional analysis of language, according to Piaget's techniques, should reveal a fall in the 'coefficient of egocentricity' or self-reference in the course of the group if therapy is proceeding satisfactorily. Serial records (ten at a time) taken from an individual's performance in the group and subjected to functional analysis can prove a good index of his progress.

Illustration from serial record.

A.B. aged 30; male; single; complains of incapacitating shyness in company and feelings of inadequacy.

Analysis of first week sample showed majority of communications directed towards conductor with high coefficient of egocentricity. Statements refer to his symptoms and feelings towards them, and feelings as a result of them. Looks bored and detached when other members are bringing up their problems.

Second analysis six months later. About 40 per cent communications now group-directed. Increase in 'mirror reactions'* and in interpretative and sympathetic responses. Some tendency to sub-grouping. Marked increase in use of 'we' and 'us'.

Third analysis ten months later. Majority of communications now group-directed. 'Mirror' and 'chain' responses* now very much in evidence. Increase in altruistic responses. (Has joined social club connected with his job. No dependency reactions.)

The swing over in the communication pattern is directly related to the technique of minimal interference on the part of the conductor. Given an authoritarian group with an active conductor, the communication patterns would show little of this dramatic change.†

Some important studies have also been carried out on the configurations in the communication pattern brought about by existing patterns of relationships. Communication linkages are plotted on a group chart as they occur during a session by an observer, arrows pointing in the direction of the communication. Between the greatest transmitter and the greatest receiver there is a gradient of transmission and reception which takes on a

* See Chapter 7 for an explanation of these terms.

† E. J. Anthony: 'Group Psychotherapy' in *Group Discussion*, ed., J. Burton, Central Council for Health Education, 1955.

configuration closely related to interpersonal feeling at the time.

The 'lines' of communication* are found to shorten with the integration of the group, as it changes from a mere collection of people, to a leader-centred group, and then to a group-centred

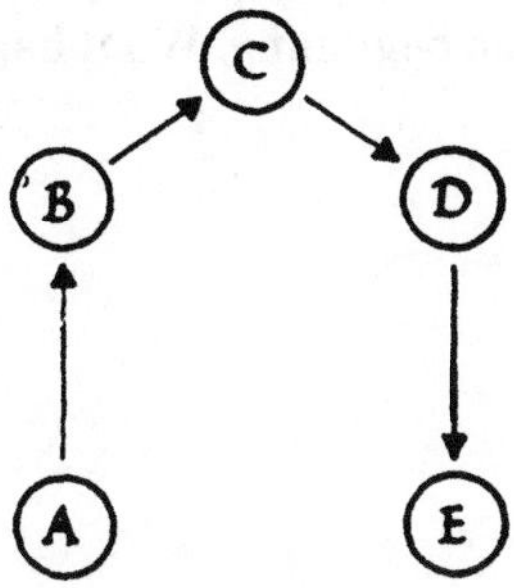

Fig. 6

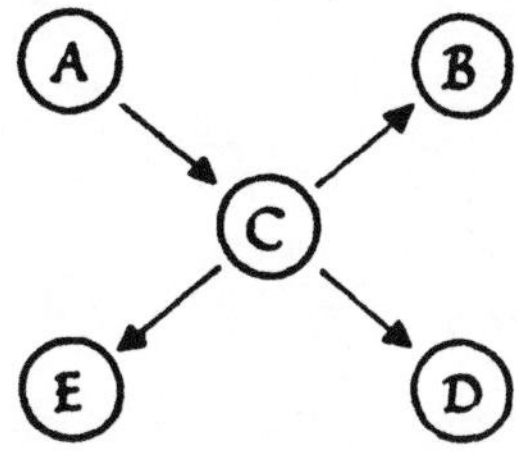

Fig. 7

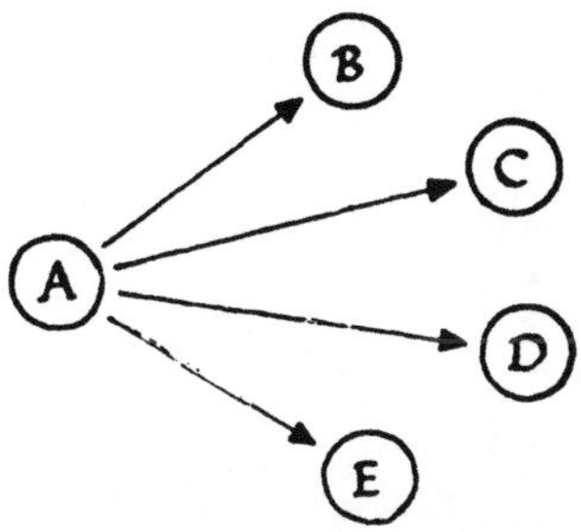

Fig. 8

FIG. 6	FIG. 7	FIG. 8
A → B = 1	A → B = 2	A → B = 1
A → C = 2	A → C = 1	A → C = 1
A → D = 3	A → D = 2	A → D = 1
A → E = 4	A → E = 2	A → E = 1
10	7	4

group. Taking the communications of member A to members B, C (Conductor), D and E, and arbitrarily giving each communication channel or arrow a unitary significance, we find the following schematic changes taking place in the course of the group:

* Alex Bavelas: 'Communicating patterns in task-oriented groups' in *The Policy Sciences*, ed., D. Lerner and H. D. Lasswell, Stanford University Press.

The 'mathematics' of communication may allow for a more scientific appraisal of such changes in communication in the course of a therapeutic group.

With the emergence of the group-centred group, the first phase of the therapeutic process is over, and the group-analytic situation is now set up. This is the end of the beginning. What happens next will depend on the group.

Chapter 5

Clinical Illustrations with Commentary

First, by way of introduction, an excerpt from a letter from a woman who is well motivated for participation in a group-analytic group:

Why I want to join a therapeutic group, and what I expect from it.

All I know at present of what goes on at a therapeutic group session is secondhand and theoretical. When I first came across Dr Foulkes' introductory book [*Introduction to Group-Analytic Psychotherapy*] I was fascinated by it to such an extent that I read it through at one sitting. Here, at last, was a 'natural' way of working out one's difficulties and problems!

When a little while before I had considered undergoing psychoanalytic treatment I had rationalized my general repugnance to having my true self laid bare by expressing doubts whether psychoanalysis was not too special, too artificial a method for me. I hardly liked the idea of being so ill that I needed the attention – hour after hour, week after week, month after month, and year after year – of a highly skilled therapist as required for full psychoanalysis. It just seemed out of proportion. I had not understood the idea that psychoanalysis aims at really changing a person. All I expected was perhaps the disentangling of a few strands in my early emotional life, and having them neatly rearranged.

Group-analysis on the other hand seemed at once to offer the proper setting for sorting out one's problems towards one's fellow men. From personal experience I knew the 'morale' value of quite ordinary discussion groups, and I had long come to the conclusion by myself that it hardly mattered what one discussed. While taking part in discussion groups and other educational activities which allowed me to 'let off steam' I had felt less unsettled. This certainly predisposed me towards group-therapy.

It has been suggested to me that this intellectual predisposition did not in any way mean that I was really serious about group-analysis. Why should I relish the idea of facing myself honestly in a group of patients any more than on a couch as in psychoanalysis? To this I can only say that I realize more and more how badly I am in need of a 'mental spring cleaning', and that I am sincere in my desire for self-inspection and purge. That is not altered by the fact that group-analysis does seem a less drastic measure, a less frightening procedure than psychoanalysis, because it is more 'real'.

I suspect myself a little of a masochistic need to lay myself bare in front of a whole group: this promises so much more than doing it just in front of one analyst. The group may also be tempting as offering greater satisfaction for my narcissistic desire to show off; I can hardly expect to impress the therapist with my miserable troubles which he must find uninteresting among the wealth of material to which he has access. Moreover, since I would pay him to listen to me, he would fail to satisfy some basic need in me (though no doubt this would in due course be analysed). With the group it is different – we are all equals, we are judged by our peers, we not only accept help, but we also give it.

Personally, I want the group to replace the sort of family circle in which there are ample opportunities for 'a good talk' with an understanding relation. Finding it hard to make such confidences to those about me, a group of people with whom I have no social contact, but which allows for the reciprocity of such personal outbursts, seems a heaven-sent solution. I have, deliberately, for years bottled up all emotions inside me, have shut myself up in myself in order not to get hurt. If I don't find an outlet soon, there must be an explosion; and yet the longer I go on isolating myself, the more impossible it becomes to find a natural outlet in everyday life. I dare not allow myself to fall in love, to find satisfaction in a worthwhile career or some other creative activity, to have a child. . . . No, I must waste my time, waste my life. I make fun of people who are ambitious and take their little selves so seriously. But perhaps my own utter lack of ambition and lack of self-respect could be but the other side of the coin?

Some things do tear at my defensive armour: a truly physical longing to 'belong' to someone, to have a child even, for the simple selfish reason of wanting someone of my own. I try not to repress such feelings as violently as I used to, but I am still far from being able to have normal relationships with other people. I think I am managing to defrost myself gradually, and I feel sure that a group could hardly fail to help me to get a clearer picture of how far I can let myself go, since I am still afraid of getting involved too deeply, of getting hurt. Why I should be such a coward in this respect I have not yet fathomed. But this fear of being humiliated, of loving one-sidedly, of making a fool of myself over a useless person – this is a very strong barrier to making friends.

The therapeutic group situation should allow me to test myself out, and discover where the basic trouble lies.

I have always managed to camouflage my lack of social relationships by finding it quite easy to be superficially friendly with people. I am then shocked to find that they carė for me more deeply than I am prepared – or able – to care for them, and I get rather 'bored' with them. My trouble has usually been to get rid of friends, men and women, and I cannot remember that I ever actively cultivated a friendship. This getting bored with people I now recognize as a self-defensive move (and it is presumably linked with making myself a bore to other people). This leads back to the question whether I am not basically too narcissistic, too self-centred, and whether I have cultivated this as self-sufficiency, as preferring my own company to that of most of my so-called 'friends', and therefore having no normal friendships, let alone satisfactory sexual affairs.

So much in a most unsystematic and rather superficial way about why I wish to join a group-analytic group.

To sum up what I expect from it: Mainly a place where I can and may openly speak about my personal problems 'amongst peers'; where I can compare my difficulties with those of other people, see in their behaviour a mirror of my own; and where, under a therapist's guidance, I can watch my own group behaviour and discover its meaning. What I picture is a sort of combined confessional, substitute for intimate talks with friends or relations, and gymnasium in which to practice my mental apparatus under supervision (assuming one would be discouraged from breaking one's neck). But more, really: a challenge to my whole attitude to life, a test of my humanity, my honesty, courage, and tolerance, and in return getting a fuller understanding of human beings, and in particular of myself. Naturally, I would hope to come out of this test not too badly, and turn out a useful member of the group.

This shows good understanding, based on favourable disposition. The writer takes well to the idea of a more active participation in a group. She gives a good account of various motivations, anxieties, reaction formations, etc. An element of flight from the overpowering exposition to a father figure can be discerned and is rationalized – as the writer says – by not needing 'the attention . . . of a highly skilled therapist . . .'.

Some Introductory Remarks on the Problems of Recording and Reporting in this Field

The value of group psychotherapy for didactic purposes highlights the need for recording the rich but ephemeral experiences of a group session. In order to study our technique, to follow specific technical problems carefully, and generally to acquire material for research purposes, we need records which enable us to study our material at leisure and over a longer stretch of time than is afforded by a single group session.

With modern sound-recording machines there is no difficulty in recording the whole session, with the agreement of its members. Although we could expect that the microphone's intrusion into their midst might upset the group's spontaneity, it is surprising how quickly it is forgotten. Sound recordings can be used in many ways. They can be played back to the group who, when confronted with what they have been saying, may react interestingly. Clearly a sound recording is far from being a complete record of a group session. We hear the voices, and what has been said, but we do not see people's facial expressions, whom they were addressing, how they sat or moved, how they hesitated before saying something or not saying it. Nor can we form any impression of those who took no audible part in the procedure at the moment and who are, as a rule, in the majority. A complete film and sound recording which would register all this is obviously far too expensive and cumbersome for ordinary clinical use, and could only be made quite exceptionally. Sound recording is the only mechanical aid we have at present. It does not give the listener the real 'feeling' of a group. Cross-talk, or laughter for instance, do not come out very clearly or naturally. It does, however, register the actual content of the session, and this is most useful. The recording can be played as often as one likes; one can go back over certain passages or episodes, and compare them with each other.

The other means of recording what goes on is by writing it down afterwards. The taking of verbatim notes during the session, be it by the conductor himself or by someone else in the group, is too distracting and interferes with the living, ever-changing process. It also gives rise to unconscious misapprehensions and misinterpretations of the situation.

Making a report from memory is open to many obvious objections – that there will be distortion, misrepresentation, biased selection, and subjectivity – which from a strictly scientific point of view must be admitted. In spite of these objections it seems possible to reconstruct fairly accurately in this way what happened in the group. Sitting down, reasonably soon after a group session, it is surprising how easily one thought leads to the next, and how fully the whole session can be reproduced. This of course takes many hours, and we never in practice find time to make such a full report. If it could be done, however, a fairly accurate and complete picture would emerge of what happened and of what was said in the group, though there would probably be some gaps, and the sequence might not always be correct.

In practice we do not aim at such completeness. Instead we ask ourselves what went on in the group, which were the most significant themes touched upon, what events were reported to the group, what reactions were observed, what observations were made concerning individual members, what changes our interventions as therapists brought about and how one theme linked up with and followed another. This record recalls to our mind a clear and comprehensive picture from which we can select, deliberately and consciously. Some events will be much condensed in our report, others which strike us as significant, either in the particular group context or in any individual's interest, will be rendered more fully. A member's attitude may be notable, or some remark, or perhaps the contrasting attitude of different members; here we obviously select what material we are putting on record. We may be interested in certain theoretical aspects, perhaps the way in which a group expresses its opposition towards the conductor, or how and in what way some observable change links up with other observations made.

Group reports such as we have in mind here are made for the group-psychotherapist's own use. They might be used for reporting to a scientific circle, or perhaps for reporting to a supervising doctor, as happens at teaching hospitals. They are straightforward reports of clinical material and, as will be explained presently, would not be suitable for publication.

Group reports need not be made by the conductor. Sometimes a member of the group may volunteer to write them down. No one so far seems to have persuaded a whole group to keep regular records, and to compare them, which should prove most interesting.

Everyone will have his own way of making such reports. We may mention here two rather different types of report by individual group members, who showed sufficient interest to write them regularly after each session. The first was a novelist who freely wove her own phantasies into the context. Though often reporting almost imaginary events, the personalities were very accurately recorded, and quite often the exact words and inflexions were caught. Some of this writer's material will be used among our illustrations, though fictitious characteristics have had to be substituted for the real ones.

The other 'reporter', a member of the same group, was a scientist. Her reports were much more accurate in the literal sense. This made them rather dry, as they did not convey anything more than the factual material remembered. Thus the writer's reports conveyed in a sense more, perhaps just because they were not aimed at being accurate at all. They bring out the atmosphere and often throw light on aspects which the more scientific report, aiming at accuracy, does not reveal, and which might also be missed in a mechanical recording. There is therefore much to be said for the more artistic, impressionistic reports when they can be had.

Only a few samples of the writer's reports can here be published, in which the actual persons are unrecognizable – we are inclined to think even by themselves. All material used for publication is changed in such a way that recognition by an outsider is impossible. These precautions necessarily involve sacrifices from the point of view of scientific accuracy, and they sometimes rob examples of the conviction they should carry to the reader. The essential elements – the principle features of any story – are maintained as far as possible, or else the whole illustration would lose its value and we would be writing fiction.

All these considerations unfortunately limit and restrict the material which can be used for illustrations. We hope, however, that they will still carry a sufficient degree of conviction. They are the best substitute we can offer for real group experience.

Our examples are chosen to show how various kinds of events occur in a therapeutic group, and to illustrate theoretical and therapeutic points made elsewhere in this book. They are selected from a great wealth of material. Sometimes various observations are brought together which in reality were seen in various groups and in different persons.

Some of the illustrations for this chapter were supplied by the writer-patient to whom we are greatly indebted. In order to preserve complete anonymity of the members concerned, any reference, however remote, to their personal circumstances, has had to be omitted and replaced by imaginary ones. Thus the material presented cannot on the whole be used for demonstration purposes.

These reports are invaluable in view of their conveying the general atmosphere of some sessions, and of their giving a lively picture of the flow of conversation in such a group. The writer, on the other hand, generously communicates some of her own, personal reactions and experiences in the group. As far as her own person goes, therefore, we have a genuine, first-hand, unreservedly valid basis for our observations. In this respect, quite particularly, our writer's contribution is of unique value.

First let us have her comments – excerpts from a letter – on the difficulties of reporting and recording, which are particularly interesting and in which she explains the situation in her own words.

Because the others enjoined it I am obliged to act as the floodlit centrepiece of a work the readers could better see if I were at liberty to make the individuals in the group true to themselves and large as life. This they would not consent to, and therefore I can best illustrate in my own person the sequence of treatment and its impact. The view I can give is therefore narrowed unfortunately; as a writer I would have enjoyed more creating the six other portraits than making my own so important.

I have never come across such stubborn rejectors of immortality as my friends in the group. Indeed it surprised me to find so vehement a reaction against the only service I could render them.

Extracts from a letter to Dr F by the same writer:

It needs no clairvoyant powers on my part to predict that I shall disappoint you over the matter of threading an account of the group into some tapestry of my own which will at the same time do justice to the original story. By the way, my condensed style owes itself in part to the fact that I expect so little patience on the part of the reader.

Last night, for example, I spent the entire session muttering 'speak bloody coward, or forever hold your peace'; apart from this I experienced vaguely a glow of anguish and embarrassment reflecting as I thought my own and radiating in turn from me to the six other members of the group. The look of sullen despair on Miss D's face endeared her to me, and I suffered for Mrs P in case she should reveal any intimate details from her life, which, however, she refrained from doing. I revolted against Mr Q's ears, grin, and glasses and his leer of intelligence. I inwardly noted that women were in general more repressed than men and wondered about the explanation, probably a social one. I heard the philosopher gravely define bullshit for Mrs P as though it were a concept of logic. Each week so far she has been stumped by a cant word and he has clarified it for her with unfailing academic tact.

Mr A earned my deepest sympathy with his account of difficulties in pursuing the object of his amorous desires, and his despair over advancing age unaccompanied by signs of progress in life. I sat in a fever of conflicting feelings through the controversy over marriage, men *v.* women, who sues and who is sued, the relative usefulness of diffidence, modesty, and bold open pursuit in the female wishing a husband and at what point pride, honesty, and fear of rebuff throw the whole box of tricks labelled technique out of the window and into the street where it properly belongs. Here I might have managed a remark or two to the effect that people who feel inadequate woo the self-confident hoping to make good the deficits in their own bravado, and on the fact that neither Miss D, nor Mrs P, nor myself felt able to take the initiative in seeking lovers. But at this point my armour began to creak, and I feared that I might fall to pieces, so I held my peace, even when you [the therapist] with a knowing and conceited smile announced that women married men, thus expressing my own inmost thoughts in all their horrid fatality.

From this you will be able to gather that the picture is blurred at the moment and I have small hopes of culling something of value to us both from the group's experiences. You need a Dostoyevsky to do the theme justice and I fear you haven't found one.

We see here, through one person's eyes, the impact of what goes on in a group. In her silent participation she shows a strong emotional involvement.

Now we shall give an example of *free-floating discussion* as reported by the same writer. It should be understood that there were at this time two conductors in the group. The report was written when one of them (Dr F) was absent, and Dr D was in charge of the group. In this example the writer shows, in her comments, her own interpersonal reactions as well as her interpretations.

I was late as an act of ineffectual revenge upon the absent Dr F.

No sooner had I sat down, with many unfelt apologies, than I became articulate and bounced into the conversation. I said my problems were like the hysterical correspondence on the back page of some weekly, and therefore I could not bring myself to air them.

'Well, why do you mind about that?' asked Miss T. (I note that a situation is blowing up between us and look forward to its eruption in puffs of hot air.) 'I have the feeling that those problems in the women's papers are very real problems, many of them are like our problems, the pity is that they should appear there where they cannot be dealt with. I don't see why you should mind.'

Dr D punctuated her comments with his morse code of nods, which I must learn to interpret more accurately than I can at present.

'I've never read such papers,' Mr K remarked, 'so perhaps you could enlighten me. I should rather like to know what these problems are they write about.'

'I expect Miss G objects to the phraseology,' Dr J surprisingly championed me, 'rather than to the problems themselves.'

I denied this which although true made me out an intellectual snob, and sidestepped: 'I can't help feeling that it's beneath one's dignity to have such trivial problems but that if one has, one can at least keep them to oneself.' Cries of indignation and protest broke out and I was moved to relate how I tremble and sniff in the company of attractive and interested men.

'That's one of my problems,' W nobly declared. 'D'you find that you begin to go to pieces when you get spiritually involved? Because that's what breaks me every time.'

'I am in pieces before I start,' said I coldly. (He would expatiate on 'necking' and I hate the word.)

Was it, Mrs F asked, that I feared men would make love to me and having met with an enthusiastic response would then lose interest and fly to others?

(Answer Yes, No, Don't know, by marking the blank spaces with a cross.)

Was it with my own or the opposite sex, Mrs M wanted to know, that I experienced this pathic unease?

'Not invariably, but on the whole I feel at ease with women,' I replied, 'coming as I do from a large family full of them it would be odd if this were otherwise. I'm not a bit used to men for we've never had any in our family.'

'Tell me, do you find that you fall in love at first sight, or is it only later when you come to know someone's character and personality? There is a difference surely.'

'First sight,' I answered with a sigh, knowing this was not the mature expression. (Indeed nowadays it would have to be first sight for I rarely get a second.)

'And what happens?' Mr K pursued with unseemly curiosity.

'What can possibly happen?' I cried with some bitterness, 'nothing happens of course.' How can people enjoy one's company if one afflicts them with one's own nervousness?

'There is mutual avoidance then?' Mr K concluded.

'Mutual,' I confirmed, blessing the dear man for that face-saving proviso. 'Men,' I explained to the group for their information, 'don't like nervy women.'

An assenting silence, a hush of affirmation greeted me. The five men bent their eyes modestly upon the floor, but Mrs M insisted that I was mistaken which was nice of her.

'I used to be like you,' Miss T suddenly commented (to my great annoyance) 'I never had any boy friends, but always girl friends (insulting, very), but now I'm perfectly at ease with men, I don't know how it happened, it just did, I'm not bothered any longer by the sexual thing, my trouble is I just sleep with whoever asks me, it has happened twice recently that I have met a man at a party and gone home with him, I didn't even know their names.'

At this Dr J sprang forward in his chair, his eyes lit up, he slapped his knee with his hand and exclaimed: 'What a bloody fool I am, I thought you were quite different, I should have known better.' For the first time he gazed upon Miss T with fond and open admiration.

'Yes,' she said, ignoring the interruption, 'I'm worried, not about the moral side of course,' she waved a disclaiming hand, 'but I don't seem able to feel anything about the man emotionally, well very little, there is some emotion because there is always some, I just sleep with him and that ends it. It doesn't give anything time to grow, that's the trouble.'

'Male psychology,' Dr J murmured sympathetically.

'But Miss T,' Mrs F cut in, 'this is surely a very recent development with you? Only eight months ago, I think, you told us you were a virgin.'

Miss T gave a pleased smile.

'Well, I admire you,' said Mrs F wistfully. 'I think you're very courageous, you must have given up a defence. But are you not frightened of the risk of it, you might have a child?'

Miss T shrugged her shoulders: 'If I have a child, well I have a child.'

(Hear, hear. Why not? The Group could adopt it.)

'Don't frighten her, don't frighten her,' Dr J protested.

(So this was the man, I told myself, who could not cheat bus conductors, O Freud. O Logical Positivists. O Tempora. O Mores. O Hell.)

'What I can't understand,' said Miss T in a tone of exasperation, 'is that anyone can make the approach and I just give them what they want. I mostly seem to have affairs with married men.'

'Oh, so you're all right then,' Dr J commented.

'No, I'm not like you in that respect,' Miss T contradicted, shaking her sleek black head, 'I'm just dying to get married.'

'Only for the security,' J pointed out half to himself, half aloud.

He turned to the contemplation of his own sexual quandary.

'These days I have to take my sex where I can find it. But if I see any question of marriage looming up, I make off on the first bus.'

We laughed. (If I ever meet Dr J on a bus instead of in the tube, I shall know that someone has proposed to him.)

Has he never entered upon any permanent relationship? asked Mrs M.

No, as a youth of twenty-one he had been ideally in love with a woman some years his senior. They had been very happy and it had lasted. As a matter of fact she was now over in England and he had to meet her this evening. Recently he had met her again after a lapse of some years. He was no longer in love with her, she had become middle-aged. (Wish he had suppressed this in view of Mrs F.) Unfortunately she still felt the same about him. In the old days she had been very beautiful and he had had a hard time defending her against his many rivals. He felt responsible for her because he had had a great influence over her and had persuaded her to interest herself in politics by reason of which she had destroyed her life.

'I wish I didn't have to go this evening,' said Dr J, fixing me with a sneering black eye, 'I should have Miss G's tremble, but I don't somehow.'

We could not offer much in the way of solution for this impasse. Men and women ought never to meet after a lapse of years. It should be forbidden by law. I myself already hate meeting people who knew me at sixteen. What will it be like in another decade or so?

A short silence fell upon the group as they digested this news and meditated other lives and other trials and tribulations.

After a suitable pause, Miss T introduced a new theme. She now complained of her lack of reserve. She respected her girl friends, she said, for being capable of reticence about themselves. She had a compulsion to share her soul with everyone she met from the moment of encounter. Either this, or she could make no relationship at all.

(*sic:* my own experience in W when I was very angry to discover my private affairs bruited abroad by all the gossip-mongers of the village and was at pains to trace the rumours to their source which turned out to be myself.)

Dr D then hunted round in the depths of his Freudian mind and produced a biological clue.

'This might link up,' he said, 'with an early disappointment over bodily production.'

(He then explained to us how infants offer their stools to adults and are upset at having this, to them, precious offering snatched away with exclamations of disgust and hurled down the drain.)

Miss T confessed that she had suffered from enuresis until late adolescence.

Mrs F said that at times during treatment she had become unaccountably constipated.

Mr K, in a low confused voice, said that his enjoyment of sex was stimulated by the idea of there being something dirty about it.

At this juncture, rather to my relief, time ran out and we adjourned.

This gives a good picture of the nature of group discussion and atmosphere. As a reaction to the absence of one of the therapists, two factors emerge: revenge on the absentee, and great liveliness. The cynicism which is notable is that of the writer, rather than a characteristic of the group. She achieves a comic effect through caricature, and pokes fun at psychology as well; for instance 'Well, I admire you . . . I think you're very courageous, you must have given up a defence' or 'Dr D then hunted round the depths of his Freudian mind and produced a biological clue . . .'.

Again, the writer here shows strong inner, silent work in relation to what is going on in the group. This factor is a very important one, though for obvious reasons is concealed.

The next example illustrates a hospital group's reaction to a change of conductor (discussed in Chapter 9, pp. 237–8), and how their reaction is expressed in indirect ways.

When Dr A left the hospital, this group of women was taken over by Dr B. Dr A and Dr B were men with very different personalities, and for this reason the handover was intentionally made rather abruptly. Dr B attended the group with Dr A for one session, during which he was introduced, and at the following session took over as the conductor.

Dr B noted at the first session which he conducted that the group carried on as if nothing had happened. They talked freely, but in a way which made Dr B feel he was being ignored. It was as if the group were *denying* the advent of their new conductor because they felt it was unpleasant. Moreover, the discussion turned on the most sombre subjects, on suicide and on incurable illness. When Dr B asked why they talked of such depressing topics, he got no direct answer, but the group then talked about how a woman should handle the problem of being abandoned by her husband.

In the subsequent sessions other patterns of reaction emerged. Attendance became irregular; a number of members consulted their family doctors and discussed this in the group; they also discussed whether they might not find a solution to their difficulties by marrying other husbands. At the same time Miss P who had had particularly strong

transference feelings for Dr A was made a scapegoat. The group concerned itself with the problem of how it should deal with bad members, much as the Chorus in *Oedipus Tyrannus* tasked itself with the duty of finding the sinner who had brought down ill luck on the city of Thebes. (See pp. 241–2.)

We see in the example the many ways in which a group deals with an intensely painful event, the loss of a conductor to whom it had been deeply attached. Its behaviour is such that it both denies and expresses that loss simultaneously, and it takes on the nature of a group symptom. We must note, however, that this symptomatic behaviour is not simply a means of evading a painful issue, it is also a means of so tempering the shock of loss that the group can survive, for the group did survive to complete its course of treatment.

The most interesting feature is the way in which an event (the change of conductor), which in this case is clear to us, reflects in remote, indirect ways: the sombre subjects discussed (suicide, incurable illness, a woman losing her husband). Then the group takes revenge by irregularity of attendance, by turning to other doctors, and even with talk of marrying other husbands! Thus they try to deal with the traumatic event by inflicting it themselves in an active role. It is also interesting to note that the member closest to the offending leader is made a scapegoat.

We shall now return to our novelist's narrative. The following pages throw light on the growing together of the group, as exemplified by her own absorption into it. Tolerance for personal remarks increases. The group is actively engaged in the analytic process, having digs at the analyst. Mrs W's reported dialogue with the writer, leading up to the statement 'I think you remind me of my younger sister' is an example of the discovery of a 'transference' reaction inside the group.

I must here correct an impression charm and distance have lent together that the group became a 'we' rather than a collection of battling 'I's' with any undue haste. Nor did I think of 'us' for many long months, nor was I much in love with the idea of being a member, but spent many an evening in sulky silence and secret criticism of Dr F and his troop of twittering bats, as in bad moods I would think of them.

Though my foullest self was at all times tolerated, the others by no means felt invariably benevolent towards me.

For example there was Mrs P's catty remark:

'You always seek small attentions from the men. I notice you always come without matches and ask them to give you a light, but you never ask the women to.'

'Yes,' said Mr M unkindly, 'the moment she came in this evening, she asked for something!'

On a subsequent occasion, the following dialogue nettled me:

MRS W: You irritate me in some ways.
SELF: In what ways?
MRS W: Well, you're limp and helpless.
SELF: What do you mean?
MRS W: Well your voice for one thing is limp and helpless. I think you remind me of my younger sister. She would leave doors open and drop forks, and there was something helpless about her, but she got away with things an awful lot because she was young and pretty.
SELF: I'm not helpless. I'm uncoordinated if that's what you refer to.
MR M: You always say you're helpless.
SELF: No.
MR M: Yes, in relation to men.
SELF: I have no men to be in relation to.
MR M: You always say you feel helpless and can't speak to them.
SELF: No, I can't listen when they talk to me.

Mrs W and Mrs P complained that I made little contribution to the problems of others in the group.

I agreed this was true and said I was sorry to be so egocentric but could see no help for it.

B tartly pointed out: 'It is not an accusation, it is being brought to your awareness.'

'Yes,' I said non-committally. (Having learnt the subtler uses of this monosyllable from Dr F himself.)

Here it will be noted that far from withdrawing into shattered silence as I would have done a few months before, I could actually speak up for myself and even take part on occasion in spirited repartee.

No one could hope for too comfortable a time in the group. Now and then, incalculably, your social mask was snatched away showing the pock-marks and superfluous hairs behind it. (If I may borrow from the awful warning language of the beauty parlours.) There was a fair measure of warmth and kindness, but it alternated with sharp sudden prods of a painful nature to self-esteem. For this reason presumably, people took pains to evolve ingenious methods of not turning up. (Which would also absolve them from the charge of moral cowardice.)

Mr I for instance was held up by a burst car tyre, leaving him stranded on the Great West Road.

Mrs M got herself knocked out by a model plane.

Mrs W became interested in mycology, which caused her to eat inedible fungi and laid her low with food poisoning.

I myself worked up some blisters to football size and could not so much as limp to the front door to hail a taxi.

Mr B made of altogether sterner, prouder stuff, quite simply forgot, at intervals, to come.

Occasionally I tried out his habit of late-coming, but in my case it was too readily spotted that this was a mere superficial need for attention, whereas with B the symptom went altogether deeper and was an integral part of his independent character.

One evening we laid bare our hopes of what grouping might do for us.

I didn't know, and only wished we could have some idea of what we really wanted.

'To like myself better,' said Mr M.

'To get on with others, to be working at full tempo,' said Mr B.

'To be able to marry again,' said Mrs M.

'To feel less frustrated,' Mrs P sighed.

'To attract lots and lots of lovely attention from men,' I made bold to declare – this I could never have enough of. Hooray!

'It could be nice,' Dr F prudently observed, 'but we aim to do a little bit more than that. You could be freer perhaps.'

'But will I ever have a sex life?' I cried in dismay.

'If not, we shall discover why' – he answered with assurance.

'Could you,' said Mr M curiously, 'have a lover now? Would you mind if he were impotent?'

'Well I would a bit,' I said, not knowing how to take him.

Mrs M told us she had opportunity for sexual intercourse on an average about once every six months and it was quite enough for her.

B here quoted some statistics he had cut from a newspaper about frequency of intercourse among married couples, and asked Dr F to confirm or refute these, which he firmly declined to do.

Mrs W said, a little ambiguously, that she would never be a whole person unless she could have a lover, but added she could not, just now, 'stand up to one'.

B suggested the analyst should prescribe us all lovers with 'to be well shaken before taken!'

Mr B's obstinate unpunctuality and Mr M's compulsion to put in an early appearance set us all talking about our respective struggles with time.

Mrs P objected to a ruling Dr F made that we should turn up within a certain time limit, or else expect to be locked out. This seemingly autocratic whim was based, he explained, on the needs of his household.

[It was in fact a concession to the locality in which this group met. F.]

Mrs P thought it proved exasperatingly how he made his own terms for us to observe. Once he had kept her waiting several minutes prior to an individual session and she had thought: he said to himself 'What does this matter? It's only Mrs P.'

Mr I agreed that he too resented being kept waiting by anyone for whatever reason.

Pending the painful, but customary, dismissal which I knew would sooner or later accrue to me from my existing employer (an advertising agent), I still could not prevent myself from arriving later and leaving earlier than other members of the office staff. (It was always a dashing experience to meet the directors of the firm on my way up the stairs some minutes after their own arrival.)

Mrs W told us that David, her son, would dawdle at his dressing and come down late for breakfast. This she felt was meant to be provoking and she was afraid that David, like her husband, would take to secret warfare. (In the case of Mr W it took the form of neglecting to carry out commissions, reading the paper at meals, and staying late at the office when upset.)

'Perhaps David resents your going to work,' said I.

Mrs W agreed that he probably did.

Mr M was loth to wake in the morning. 'There's a grey mechanical routine,' he said, 'that goes around being me. Why should I put it in action?'

Mr B could not wake. The problem was serious. He might lose his job by failing to get there. When he had rejected, on one ground or another, every suggestion as to aids to waking, Mr I recommended him to try marriage. 'Then you will easily get up in the morning,' he thought.

Dr F reflected how perverse it was that attitudes towards time influenced people so much throughout life.

Mr I supposed it had to do with early potting duels between our mothers and our infant selves.

Mrs W said mothers were too powerful, no one should be given such a burden of power; she thought home influence should be countered as much as possible by nursery schools and other counter power zones.

I kept up a bored silence as always when the others talked of their families, feeling jealous at having none. B said there we were back on the potting level where we all belonged.

I thought such interpretations very queer and by no means accepted them.

The whole passage shows the theme of neurotic difficulties with time (punctuality, etc.) displayed in a typical variety of ways. Acting out – somebody over-punctual, somebody always late –

protest against the physician's tyranny, autocratic privileges. This is paralleled by behaviour in life itself.

Members give, at the same time, their different interpretations of these neurotic difficulties, at first convergent ones, later divergent ones, as well as their defensive reactions to these. Mrs W's reference to her child is a good example of a kind of interpretation by inference, which may be conscious, but is very often made unconsciously in a group. The serious and apparently remote symptom of 'not waking up in the morning' betrays one of its roots by being brought up in this context. Characteristically its bearer protests against the 'potting level' mentioned by another member. The writer herself likewise rejects these 'queer interpretations'. However, her very next remark about her writing inhibition is revealing ('so small was my output').

Difficulties with work often recurred as themes in the discussion.

Whatever job I was doing, and I did a great many, I never felt rightfully occupied – if on the other hand I turned to writing that did not seem to suit me either – so small was my output and so great my disinclination to attempt it.

Mrs M accused me of working with contempt (for both work and employer). This, she said, made her 'boil with fury'. Later she admitted feeling very contemptuous towards her own chosen occupation, as she would really have preferred to read law and become a barrister and rather despised herself for being a mere handmaiden of the courts.

Mr M, who was temporarily fretting behind the bars of a news agency, remarked how odd it was that he had always worked more willingly for women than for men.

On which Mr I commented: 'Excuse my crudeness, but women don't have penises.'

Mrs W, who occasionally gave lectures, found it difficult to speak at public meetings. The former she could do quite easily because it was 'all prepared beforehand', but the latter made her heart beat and thoughts parch up.

Four among us were addicted to writing.

Mrs W negatively, in that she half wished to write a book, but was nauseated at the idea of exposing herself to the public.

(We argued here as to whether expose or reveal was the more apt term and everyone seemed to perceive different shades of meaning in either.)

Mrs P half-heartedly; the chief librarian at the public library had expressed interest in her work, so it was, she supposed, query, valuable. Anyway she had been writing it for so long that it acquired power over her and she dared not lay it aside. (There were many desperate moments in our time together when Mrs P's biography was threatened with dereliction, but somehow it always survived to put out new chapters.)

Mr M despondently; he had been invited to produce a short work on the golden age of English eccentrics which he said, having once accepted the offer, he had failed to tackle for some months. He claimed that so far it had turned out to be dull and shapeless as a Wellington boot. On the other hand he did not take up B's kind offer to read it; as he thought B could not judge its literary value.

Myself, mythically, in that the thought of writing and discussion about it seemed to occupy me far more than writing itself.

Mrs P could not produce more than a page or two each working day.

I call that – said I wistfully – proliferating. By my standards you are on the way to greatness.

The group discussed what value could be put on work. The criterion of work, said I, was payment in cash.

Certainly not, said M and B, shocked by this callous definition.

Mr I advised us to go on the assumption we were third-rate and thus save ourselves unnecessary *sturm und drang*.

Yes, but – protested B – you're talking to people who aren't yet persuaded they're third-rate. We're still on our way to discovering that.

Here, now, are some excerpts from different reports by the same writer. A number of cross-sections have been selected, showing the same group at different periods, and throwing light on the slow development of the group.

For some months our meetings were characterized by an atmosphere of watchfulness, weariness, and suspicion. We eyed and sniffed each other like strange dogs connected by several different collars to a master leash. Our hackles would rise at the least thing, then we would snarl and bare our teeth, wait for the word of command from Dr F and lie down again uneasily together. (The exception to this was Mrs W who seemed friendly and well-disposed from the start, with the effect that she was for some time the best-liked character among us.)

For instance Mr B rebuked Mr M: Is there anything you don't know about? You're like a walking encyclopedia.

That's more interesting at any rate than being a policeman without authority, which is how you impress me – he rudely replied.

(By now it had become clear that Mr M disliked the pedant in Mr B and Mr B was irritated by the dilettantism of Mr M.)

In an effort to break down my invariable silence, I was asked why I did not wear my specs, and what were my reasons for sitting a little apart.

'Oh, so that you can't see me,' I answered.

Mrs M here remarked: 'You seem to look at the women when you speak, but never towards the men.'

'Without my glasses,' I said tartly, wounded by his remark, 'I can't see either.'

It transpired that Mr I had always wanted to wear specs to give himself importance.

Mr M suggested he should buy frames and have lenses put in of plain glass.

Mr B detested wearing his specs, because it made people come too close. 'I want to push them away,' he said.

About my recent experiences, when pressed, I found I could say very little and even that I managed to present in terms of custardpie comedy; after which I grew offended with everybody for laughing. The others could not understand why I felt so afraid, or how being among them represented safety and a barrier against importunate spirits.

'If someone came to you at midnight and walked through the wall, would not that be frightening?' I asked.

'No, interesting,' Mr B said.

Mrs W and I agreed mutually that we could not spend a night alone in a haunted house, and she added that the supernatural alarmed her because of the surprise and shock involved in meeting ghostly beings.

'Can I speak now, or have you a problem to solve,' was one of my favourite gambits; then having secured attention to myself, I could think of nothing to talk about.

'How can group-analysis help you?' I asked Dr F in despair.

'How can it not,' he stoutly averred, 'if you let it.'

I felt he had rather a bee in his bonnet.

None of us quite knew at this early stage what was expected of us; it was seldom, as happened in later proceedings, that someone initiated a theme which would be taken up and developed by the others. Although we turned to Dr F he denied us instruction, and so we groped along our narrow confessional ledge each with his or her own awkwardness, hoping to avoid a too sudden precipitous drop into reality.

Being somewhat prudish in defence against my basic coarseness, I always feared the talk might turn rude; as I knew one had, in analysis, to speak freely about matters which were usually taboo. I was afraid that the three other women, all of them a few years older than myself, might mention their sex lives in precise detail, which idea much unsettled me. At the same time, I wanted analysis to be frank and kept resolving to say something that would shock, without however succeeding in doing so.

Mrs W courageously initiated what seemed to me the first awkward confession by admitting an impulse to eat corpses and hopefully asking us what it could mean.

We did not, or dared not, know and left it to Dr F to point out a possible connexion between necrophily and coprophily upon whose borders Mrs W perilously stood. (Or so I felt, torn between pity and admiration for her frankness.) Mrs W, it should be here explained, was not much in contact with corpses as a rule but occasionally came across them (through a view of the dissecting labs) when she visited her pathologist husband at the hospital where he worked.

Soon following upon this came a slight thaw in the atmosphere. We were beginning to trust each other a little. Someone even let fall a complaint about a parent, and another criticized a husband. Mr I volunteered, about his wife, 'she's a very tolerant girl, we don't like each other much as people.' When asked why he had married her, he said it was through 'lack of will-power'. 'How,' said Mrs M wistfully, 'did she get you?' 'Do men marry women, or women marry men?' Mr I asked Dr F, adding scornfully, 'I'm asking *you* as the only trained psychologist here.' 'Women always say,' said Dr F, grinning from ear to ear in a most annoying way, 'I married him.' 'Old peacock,' I murmured to myself, 'just what *you* would think!'

This silent contempt alternating with equally inarticulate affection was very characteristic of my feelings towards people in general and Dr F in particular.

However I believed I was well-disposed and even amiable, not to say mild and timid, so that when Mr B suddenly rounded on me, I was full of injured surprise.

'You just sit there,' he said, 'looking tense and bored. You remind me – sorry to have to say this – of a snake that now and then spits venom. You don't attack us individually, but I've watched you, when things get lively and you think it will pass unobserved, striking out blindly against us all!'

'Because I am too cowardly,' I meekly answered, while feeling chaotic and trying to muster some thoughts, 'to attack individuals openly, do you suppose?'

'No,' Mr B snapped, 'I don't!'

Mr M thought I was like a trapped animal snarling and spitting from its cage.

Mrs W could see his meaning.

As yet Dr F did not.

While I was still dazed from the above observations, Mr B went on to describe Mr M as looking black.

'He does not look black,' I defended him, 'the shadows on his face make it seem so.'

Mrs W said: 'I don't think Mr M looks black, but he seems to me a person who might sulk and hold on to grievances for a long while.'

'That is so,' Mr M assented.

Here Mr I asked rather shyly:

'Do I look black? How would you say I looked?'

'White,' B cuttingly assured him, 'pure white, white as chalk, white as cream cheese.'

Mr I glowered reproachfully and huddled in his chair. He said nothing more after this.

For weeks I was stunned by Mr B's ringing blows. I missed an evening's sport or two from pique and alarm, but was disarmed on my return to find Mr B much upset by his having been accused of driving me away. He was however less concerned with my feelings, than to discover why it upset him to learn this.

In a short while however, I found myself slapping everyone's face, just as B had mine.

'I don't like Mrs W's hats,' I said, or, 'I's voice and his canting monotonously in textbook Freud makes him awfully boring to listen to. Mrs P's and Mrs W's marriages sound pretty dull to me, anyway I think you all dull sometimes. Dull, stuffy, and bourgeois, just like myself, O God, why had I to come here in the first place. I wish you wouldn't all listen so reverently to Dr F whenever he brings out a sentence. And when I think the whole aim of life is to unite one pissing, sweating body with another in order to make more of the same, and they all become nauseous gases, I can't think why we bother to better ourselves or what we hope to get out of ever going in for this.'

To my surprise this verbal tantrum was greeted with a short silence, followed by kindly questioning. I had never before spoken truthfully without reprisal.

Mr M, who had, he apprised us, listened throughout for undertones of emotion, asked me to criticize him too.

'Oh you,' I said, trying to invent something, 'I despise you for not being able to come out with your feelings except on paper.' (Shortly before he had confessed to keeping a diary.)

'What about me,' Mr B asked. 'What do you think of someone who can't even get that far, can't even set down his feelings on paper.'

'He wants you to criticize him,' Dr F explained.

'I can't,' I said baffled, 'he doesn't make sense to me.'

'Well I am from Glasgow at that,' said Mr B, 'not one of the natives here, come to think of it. After all, in some places even the chap from the next village is looked on as a foreigner.'

These passages illustrate some characteristic stages in the development of the group. They show first the tendency to put the conductor into the centre and to expect instruction from him. He is reluctant. The group then shows reactions of ambivalence towards him.

The gradual relaxing of censorship can be discerned. This is accompanied by a greater ease in discussing awkward themes. There are also far more frank personal remarks – unpleasant ones, too – as an expression of releasing the more conventional social barriers.

There are signs that the group is becoming more active in the analytic process, for instance when they accuse Mr B of having driven the writer away (correctly, as we know from her) which shows that her absence had become a topic of discussion, and the reasons for her absence had been investigated by the group.

Here we would like to give an example or two of the patient's conflicts as expressed in his various relationships, at various stages.

Mr B is middle-aged. He lost both his parents when he was very young, and was brought up, as an only child, by his grandmother. His grandmother was an extremely warm mother substitute to him, and he naturally became very attached to her and had a deep affection for her.

The grandmother tried hard to make up the loss of his parents, and was quite especially lenient and understanding with him. This as we shall see shaped his character. (We might note here *en passant* that grandparents as a rule are less ambivalent, less 'hot' as it were, than parents towards their children.)

Mr B remained somewhat self-centred, narcissistic, and is sensitive to criticism. He has been content, as his doctor put it, to drift along the easy way, and did not develop much drive.

He married a woman who has very close ties with her own mother, which Mr B feels threatens to estrange his wife's love. He is suspicious and jealous, and sometimes he encourages his wife to be with other men and then watches jealously how far she goes. Or he provokes arguments with her to test out how she reacts. In their more intimate relationships he likes her to take the initiative; this again gives him reassurance that he is really loved.

Perhaps we can break in here to explain that these observations are the outcome of the study and the information which the doctor gains from treating the patient. It is not unlike watching a play and gradually getting to know a character's story and dilemma.

Certain features have become very clear during this treatment.

Mr B was the undisputed object of his grandmother's admiration, he had her very much alone to himself, had all her love and care. He cannot bear a situation where another person, like his mother-in-law, comes into his life, although we may suspect that – unconsciously – he hopes that his mother-in-law could take the place which his grandmother had in his childhood, and that she would be his 'ideal person'. This might account for the friction in his relationship with his wife.

In this situation in which he is constantly testing, tempting, and provoking his wife, he wants to be loved; in that sense he wants his wife to take the initiative. In the same sense his doctor reported that he wanted his wife to look after the money; she even drives him and does all the planning. This is a very characteristic example here of wanting something in one way and resenting it in another: he does resent being directed. In other words he displays a conflict, which he has in himself, between himself and his wife, has strong resentments against his wife for being the more able, and is angry with himself for not doing things for himself. There is therefore this counter-current in him which makes him want to show his wife (as well as himself) that he *can* do things.

We see here how the patient's original family situation – his relation to his grandmother – is displayed again in his marital situation, the troubles in which are central and significant for his seeking treatment.

Now let us go a step further and see how the treatment situation itself is drawn into this same conflict of feeling. Having to come for treatment and to ask for psychiatric advice is a narcissistic hurt to him. He therefore presents the same conflict all over again: he wants to be told, to be helped by the therapist, but at the same time he resents having to be told. He thus has the same conflict towards the physician; moreover, he resents the fact that his wife does not also need treatment. Like so many people, he feels that having to come for psychiatric treatment is an admission of a personal failing, and he would like his wife to take her share of blame, as it were, in this failing.

This simple example shows us how a relationship in childhood reflects in the patient's life, in the conflict which makes him have to undergo treatment, and again in the way the treatment situation is seen. It shows us the significance of relationships which contain the relevant conflicts being carried on from one situation to the other, and being re-established there, even to the treatment situation between himself and the doctor (in this case in the individual treatment situation).

Another similar example:

Mrs O, an actress, suffers from constricting feelings in the throat which she is afraid may interfere with her career. These feelings are accompanied by feelings of anxiety before and during performances.

She is thirty, and married. It turns out that she has frequent quarrels with her husband. It also emerges that her constrictive feelings in the throat developed when her mother was seriously ill, and Mrs O feared she would be left 'all alone and in the middle of nowhere' if the mother should die. She also has feelings of guilt because she had in fact unconscious wishes that her mother should die.

We may note here that there is a significant conflict between being dependent and being independent as expressed in being left alone by the mother, and not being able to be left alone. This is expressed in an ambiguous feeling about the possibility of the mother's death.

Her very profession as an actress is the outcome of her striving for independence. She resents her mother's over-solicitous attitude, for which she has a very good name, 's-mothering'.

Here we see in a nutshell one of the meanings of the constrictive feeling in her throat.

In childhood terms she is somewhere sexually tied up with her father. She used to like to dress as a boy, says she always wanted to be a boy and felt that to be a girl was shameful and an admission of insignificance. She felt it was very 'unfair' when she first menstruated and felt ashamed of her breasts when they first developed. These are very characteristic feelings shared by many girls. In her particular case they are bound up with her relationship with her father.

Her doctor makes an interesting remark here: she does not like men to approach her, not even her husband. She feels men are not to be trusted.

When Mrs O was seven, her younger sister died. This sister was actually prettier than herself, and she remembers feeling jealous. The older girl brought the infection into the house, and her father blamed her for being the cause of her sister's death. This is significant even if the father never said this – we cannot check whether this is Mrs O's phantasy or not, but it is of importance in either case, and reflects her own self-reproaches. Even while under treatment she still showed much emotion and guilt feelings when talking of these events, which probably originated in part from wishes arising in the normal course of sibling jealousy to have her sister out of the way.

In her present life she has become very fond of a woman friend who reminded her very strongly of her sister. We have learned to take such superficial conscious remarks as 'she reminds me of my sister' as an indication for deeper unconscious identification. We can therefore assume here that the emotions and deeper feelings about this woman friend are what we call 'transference', i.e. they have the power to carry with them unconscious unresolved conflict into a new situation. This is characteristic of transference. This is an example of a patient 'transferring' in life, without any treatment situation, as so often happens. All she is conscious of is that the friend reminds her of her sister. She says 'I mother her and feel responsible for her' – for instance when she was making a cup of tea for her friend and was asked what she was doing she said, 'I'm making a cup of tea for my sister.' It is thus quite clear that this friend is a substitute for her sister, and that she now, in her own language, 's-mothers' this friend.

In her childhood relationship to both her parents, she always felt she was intruding between her father and her mother. There were frequent parental arguments, and her mother did accuse her of breaking up things between them when she was a child. She sums it up by saying that her mother did not love her father, but at the same time the mother did not want him to look at anyone else, not even her [our patient].

The mother ran down the father, said that men were terrible, and must not be trusted. [As noted before, this idea of 'not trusting men' has become the patient's own, and she puts this back on to her mother.] She expressed phantasies in treatment that her father might kill her mother.

This story shows a patient who complains of a nervous feeling which as likely as not might be considered a physical affliction (namely a constriction of the throat) which is closely connected with the patient's work. The constrictions disturb her in connexion with her performance, and this performance itself is under conflict in relation to dependence or independence, and this dependence or independence is closely bound up with her mother.

This is a very good example for the reader who is not so familiar with psychiatric investigation and observation of how behind the bodily symptom there is a mental conflict. It is clear that the mother's illness and the patient's fears and wishes concerning it, together with her feelings of guilt at her mother's death, have provoked this symptom, since the attitude towards the mother is basic for this conflict over dependence and independence. The patient has in this case a very good way of expressing the double meaning of her symptom when she refers to her mother's 's-mothering' her.

Although the patient's relationship to her father shows certain typical and classical signs of disturbance as well, these are more apparent in her relationship with her younger sister, which exemplify particularly clearly how feelings can be 'transferred' from a relationship in childhood to one in the immediate present.

Mrs O also has a difficult situation in her marriage. It turns out that her husband is 'the sort of man' her mother would have wished her to marry. According to her she succeeded in marrying her mother's ideal, a person whose character is the very opposite of that of her father.

On one level then Mrs O has married an ideal father. On another level, however, the patient wishes her husband to be an ideal mother to her. She expects the same support from him that her mother gave her. As is so often the case, the husband cannot fulfil the idealized phantasy hopes which his wife, mainly unconsciously, wishes to gratify through him.

Because the husband cannot give her the support and total security which she demands from him as a mother ideal, she feels deserted and feels that she cannot rely on him. The unfortunate husband, with good reason as we can see, but from another point of view quite wrongly, treats the patient as a child, which she greatly resents. The patient is in an acute conflict of dependence–independence. Anything which makes her feel her dependence is resented, as she must be independent. At the same time she wants to be dependent and to be made secure. The husband inevitably disappoints her, because he cannot be an ideally dependable person, and she cannot tolerate the thought that she depends on him. If he treats her as a child he responds to part of her need, for that is how she actually behaves towards him, but her wish to be a child is also the very thing she fights so hard against. He disappoints her firstly by not being the completely dependable superman, a male version of the idealized mother, whom she desires him to be, and then having failed to fulfil this idealized role, he treats her as a child, which to her is adding insult to injury.

This kind of misunderstanding in which unconscious wishes are only too well understood by the participants is very characteristic of many neurotic conflicts and many marriages. The patient now resents being treated as a child who cannot look after herself, and she feels that her husband treats her as an incapable and unintelligent person. This recapitulates for her the attitude she felt her mother had, the very attitude she resents and speaks about most. This naturally makes for a bad relationship, tense, hostile, and leading to quarrels. In the family situation she identifies herself with her eldest son of eight in his feelings with his father. When her husband becomes irritable with her son, for example, she shouts at him and explains that she actually feels herself to be in her son's place and that she feels his resentment against the father as if it were her own.

We can imagine without much difficulty the rest of the picture, and the accumulative deterioration of the marriage relationship.

We see again in this example how the early family constellation repeats itself and reflects in later constellations, and is shaping them in ways which must lead to severe conflict. We can also see very clearly the effects of transference from both parents, from the idealized mother on to the husband, and from the younger sister on to the friend.

The following example gives an idea of information gained purely from group sessions, and the story itself is one which has many typical features.

Mrs M's doctor finds it worth reporting that Mrs M's father often drank to excess and this had at times got him into trouble with the police. Mrs M is a young woman who – like many others – feels rather repelled by her father. She dislikes his physical presence and also hearing him talk. She says that her mother suffered on his account in the past, and the patient now feels full of hate and resentment about this. She made the interesting statement that she hates to see her husband and her father together, because she is afraid that her husband might become like her father.

Such feelings and apprehensions can be taken as indications that somewhere underneath there is another attitude towards the father, one of being attracted. Or we might put it differently and say that the aversion is in part a defence against unconscious feelings of attraction. Her apprehension that her husband might become like her father is thus justified, if it is understood to refer to her own, inner, psychic reality.

This patient, like the last one we described, is very close to her mother. The mother takes care of her, dusts and hoovers for her, takes her home with her, and accompanies her to the hospital. At this stage of the group treatment she has said little about her elder brother and her elder sister. This may be because they are not particularly important in her life; but it may also mean that they are significant, but that the patient is cautious and hesitant about recounting reminiscences, feelings, or experiences of them. In the latter case the patient is liable to transfer her attitudes to her brother and sister, in the way we have explained, on to the other members of the group. She therefore has no particular need to talk about them. She did say a lot about a younger sister who had had some infectious illness which the patient had shared, and who was also very nervous. The patient felt she was responsible for these nervous difficulties of her sister.

The whole constellation of this case reminds us forcibly of the case we had just described from individual observation. The remarkable features in this constellation are the closeness of the mother, and the feeling of having done harm to a younger sister. As in the first case there were marital quarrels. The husband was extremely kind to the patient, he avoided arguing or otherwise upsetting her, took her to the hospital in his car, and waited patiently until the group session was over. Here again we find a close attachment to the husband, reminiscent of Mrs M's mother relationship. Nevertheless, there were quarrels between this couple, and Mrs M somewhat resented her husband's calm attitude, and felt guilty whenever she had been bad-tempered with him. Mrs M was also very strict towards herself, and showed – at this time – a marked reaction to any mention of unfaithfulness in the group.

It was now observed that a certain theme made its appearance in the patient's behaviour in the group. She used at this stage to sit near the door and she became fidgety and ill at ease, wanting to be well-placed to leave the group quickly if that became necessary. She had developed from a state of very active participation, from being a popular member of the group, into this state of apprehension.

This case shows, in so far as reported here, only individual information. This should be compared to the preceding case which is similar. It will be seen that the information gained about the personal life of the present patient compares well with the previous one, although of course the therapist did not in any way concentrate his attention on this patient and her particular story.

We pass on to another type of observation, *illustrating interaction between two members of a group* which results in what is known technically as 'acting out'.

Mr Y and Miss Z are two members of a mixed group of seven people. They have shown great interest in one another and have clung together from the beginning. At the time when the observations were made this had taken a more dramatic form.

It had been observed that Mr Y and Miss Z talked more to each other than to the rest of the group, and they sometimes stayed in the hospital for a social evening and danced together. After group meetings they began to travel together on the same bus.

One lived on the south bank and the other on the north bank of the river, the two districts being connected by a particular bridge.

Of late, Mr Y has improved considerably in relation to the street fears for which he had come for treatment, but his fear of crossing the street was now replaced by a fear of crossing the bridge!

In the group he had become aware of his feelings and able to express them more freely and had gained insight into some of the causes of his fears. At the same time it was not at all clear to him why he had improved nor why the bridge had become the focus of his anxiety.

About three sessions prior to the time of this report Mr Y stated again that he was much better, and could even travel on a bus with his children to the shops and take them out. One session later, he said he felt as bad or worse than he had ever felt and at the end of that session he approached the therapist declaring himself rather desperate about his situation. The doctor however encouraged him to deal with this matter by bringing it up during the next meetings of the group. At this next session Miss Z volunteered a statement which turned out to be a sort of confession made with the consent of Mr Y.

Miss Z recalled the fact that the doctor had asked all members to bring up in the group any experiences or incidents which occurred between group meetings and especially those which involved other members of the group. She now told the group that Mr Y had felt very upset after the last meeting and had asked her to leave the bus with him and to accompany him across the bridge almost as far as his house. In actual fact she had had to stand by until he was safely inside his front door.

At this point Mr Y exclaimed that he felt that Miss Z was the only woman who really understood him. She did not tell him to 'pull himself together' or that 'there was nothing to worry about' or that he 'must just do it and go ahead down the street and not mind' and so on. She really understood.

It was becoming very clear that Mr Y in a sense felt himself to be in love with this girl and that this created a very difficult situation, which he expressed by saying he did not know what to do. ('Crossing the bridge!')

An interesting observation here, and one which is often made, is that the group was much better aware of what was going on than the conductor, although he himself was not exactly surprised by the turn of events and had suspected some development of this kind. The rest of the group however were fully aware of this developing relationship.

At this stage nothing more had occurred between them but nevertheless Mr Y exclaimed 'What am I going to do? It is terrible.'

The group was curious to know if this type of help were really expected from them, whether they ought to advise one another and what steps the therapist would take. Interestingly enough, some time later Mr Y again asked the girl to take him home and at the same time he came to the hospital accompanied not by his wife but by his – mother.

Somewhat later the meaning of Mr Y's acting out became clear to him. His fear of crossing streets was, as is common in such cases, an unconscious fear of the temptations of the street, and camouflaged a conflict between his wishes to indulge in sexual promiscuity and his fear of punishment if he did so. During the short individual treatment he had had before joining the group, his doctor had pointed out to him this connexion between his fear of crossing streets and the temptations of the street. Mr Y did not accept the doctor's interpretation but shortly after this individual treatment he had an affair with an elderly woman. As the group treatment progressed Mr Y suddenly understood that his street fear was really connected with sexual temptation, and this insight came to him at the same time as his feelings towards Miss Z broke through, arousing very strong feelings of guilt since he unconsciously equated going home with Miss Z to committing adultery with her.

This account raises the very important question of how far this type of 'understanding' which develops between people and which stands, as this case well demonstrates, for a deeper emotional bond between them, a kind of love, is desirable or undesirable.

At this point we only wish to point out how very important it is that the transference character of such events be clearly understood not only by the conductor but also by the other patients in the group. We know these transference feelings very well from individual psychoanalytic treatment. The concentration of feelings on the analyst which occurs must be used to further the analysis and must not be exploited. The handling of this concentrated transference feeling, which the analytic situation evokes, forms an essential part of psychoanalytic treatment. So long as the group analyst and the psychoanalyst respectively fully understand the transference character of both the affection and the hostility directed against them, all is well.

It also happens quite frequently that certain reactions of the same character are transferred to persons outside the therapeutic situation. This is called 'acting out', and forms an important technical problem. The therapist endeavours, by the analysis of such relationships in the therapeutic situation, to develop the patient's insight and so to utilize such 'acted out' relationships for the purposes of the treatment. By analysing it he dissolves the relationship and renders it innocuous as a life experience. In this he is generally but not always successful.

The observation, which we are presenting, provides an example of acting out in the group situation. Two distinct and interesting differences between the group and the individual situation may be mentioned. The first is that acting out, which, involving strangers, occurs right outside the therapeutic situation in the individual setting, here, in the group setting, occurs inside the therapeutic situation itself. If in our example Mr Y or Miss Z had been in individual treatment, the other partner would be totally *outside* control and observation. In this case both parties are *inside* the same therapeutic situation and therefore their whole relationship can be seen from both sides and their interaction can be made the object of investigation and of treatment. From this angle at least the group gives us a better chance of studying and treating patients who act out.

The second point is that the relationships which form between patients in a group lend themselves readily for acting out (dramatizing) conflicts. The technical answer to this is to analyse continuously these multiple relationships between two or more members of a group, and so to further the group's understanding and insight with regard to the special character of such occurrences. While one or two members may be in too acute an emotional state to be amenable for the moment to an analysis of their reactions, the others can watch events in a more detached way, similar to that of the therapist, and by so doing can acquire deep insight. As a result those who have watched are quicker to recognize the significance of their own reactions, when they in turn are emotionally involved. In addition, active participants are often more ready to accept the comments of other patients on the nature of an acted-out relationship than the comments of the professional therapist.

We now come to another example of transference, once again from the pen of our imaginative artist-writer. This time we shall get a glimpse of how the situation appears to the patients in a group setting, though unfortunately for reasons of discretion we cannot make the presence of the group as strongly felt as in fact it was.

This report brings out several interesting points very clearly:

(1) The group members as rivals and, on another (more primitive) level, the whole group as an object or a person.

(2) The modifying and correcting influence of other members' reactions, e.g. on p. 108 when the other members think her

'favoured', or later, her observations of similar reactions by the other group members: 'They consoled and corrected me.'

(3) The direct transference with strong sexual conflict, and its illusionary strength.

(4) The growing insight into the patient's own feelings by herself.

Dr F (still in my dreams) more and more gave up his own personality, so far as it existed for me, and took to wearing my father's distinctive clothes. He even painted a portrait, drab and sugary it was I noted, peering through a skylight into the studio from which as usual I was shut out. 'You would rather,' I told the dream figure, 'paint mediocre pictures than spend time with me, old, nasty, fool!'

I found it none too easy at first to digest the idea of being in love once with my father. It seemed preposterous, though turning it round and round I was able to see something in it. As Mr B sagely remarked: 'I could never understand how I was supposed to be in love with my mother at two or three years old because I can't have been biologically equipped to sleep with her – but now I see it is all rather subtle.' Anyway, I certainly seemed to be in a dependent child–father relationship to Dr F, my dreams and phantasies, interpreted, all showed an exclusive preoccupation with a father figure and the feelings I had of being continually rebuffed did not square up with the analyst's kindness to me, but rather were based on unreasonable claims for an all-attentive love of which I had once felt cheated. So much with his help I could learn and see, though the seeing alone did not always succeed in keeping my griefs and angers at bay.

Sometimes I airily permitted myself to believe that he too was infatuated with me, but when in this yet more fatuous mood, when every sign from a cordial 'Good evening' to 'Would you mind turning on the lights?' corroborated the phantasy, I was liable to weave into moods of disgust and contempt and quickly replaced my idol on his pedestal.

For, here again to quote Mr B: 'If anyone loves me I despise them. I think I'm so ugly there must be something wrong with them to want me.'

Dr F, poor man, could do no right. Strangely enough – from my point of view – the women began to round on him, accused him of favouring me most, said that whatever I had to say was treated as interesting and important, that he neglected their problems in favour of mine. This seemed to surprise him almost as much as myself. On the one hand there was I nagging him by the hour for failing to love me enough; on the other hand there were the rest of the group charging him with undue partiality.

I for my part felt doubly exasperated; for not only did the others refuse to show solidarity over his neglect of me, they were even becoming unfriendly for fear I was the loved one.

To return to the vexed subject of Mrs M, my rather touching *bête noire* and partner in foolish misery. I kept harping on how much I minded her and how much above all I minded her getting special attention.

Dr F at last said: 'Are you really so jealous and childish that you can't bear to share me with the others who need me as much as you do?'

The truth in this remark stung me so much that for days I wandered about in a queer confusion of resentment, unable to give any attention at all to the tasks of daily life. Even a word of earned criticism from the coveted source of love and admiration would stretch me out flat as a punch in the nose.

'You are pushing all my buttons,' I petulantly cried.

'Those buttons are the one thing I want to, I am going to push,' cruelly replied the great man. [The reader will allow for poetical liberty in the remarks attributed here to the therapist.]

Dr F tried to compare me to a disgruntled child.

'So would you be disgruntled,' I pointed out, 'if people dropped scorpions in your milk.'

'Well, but why must you stay a child?' he said, 'you don't seem to have liked it much when you were one.'

He tried explaining to me that this possessive love was akin to the infant's desire to possess the breast completely. It was a great shock, he insisted, when infants discovered there were other objects in the world besides the breast. 'Like Mrs M,' I murmured defiantly, 'and psychiatric groups. Oh well, I can enter into their feelings, poor little brutes.'

In spite of this being therapy as opposed to actual experience (the distinction is the world's, not mine), I felt myself thwarted in love, though Dr F firmly repeated that I was no great tragic figure, just rather luckier than most of my friends who had to settle their conflicts and problems as best they could without expert help. I could never have suffered him to be right in this judgement were it not for the unreasonable reactions so clearly presented by Mrs P and Mrs M. They consoled and corrected me. However it was, as he said, a 'funny kind of love', and took the form of wishing him dead, finding fault with him, and generally airing many other savage impulses, hitherto unsuspected. For some reason it was easier to express hate than loving or sexual feelings. Dr F seemed startled and a little taken aback on learning how full of hate I was, since when the group first called me 'serpent' he had not shared their view. Now he began to observe that my face contorted with malice when Mrs M was present and said he felt sorry for anyone burdened with so much hatred. With a prod here, and a push there, we began little by little to uncover the anatomy of my hatred, and very complex it proved to be indeed.

To begin with the simpler nursery clues and those that came easiest to light all centred round my unhappy father. (Unhappy in the sense that he had not the least wish or intention to play such a damaging part in my development.) I often lost all perspective on my situation and found it impossible to decide which of my feelings were contemporary, and which belonged to an earlier phase. Hence I was often made wretched by not being all-in-all to Dr F and could never quite accept that he was not a present frustration but an index to all that had gone before. The pleasure of meeting and sadness of parting were like two hands on a clock. This time-keeping made up my inner world. The outer was still very trying and I tended to slither about in it; I still could not measure the relationship between the two but knew that it altered imperceptibly as I made progress.

In the following example we wish to illustrate the patterns of *various treatment situations* which might be used to deal with a case and we have illustrated these opposite.

The patient in this case, whom we will call Miss K, came with a problem in which other members of her family were involved and which could not be understood without reference especially to her father and mother. In real life, therefore, the problem was one involving father, mother, and daughter which we illustrate in Fig. 9.

It was, however, the daughter who came for treatment, and the first individual treatment pattern is illustrated in Fig. 10 in which the therapist and the daughter (= patient) participate. Soon, however, the therapist becomes aware of the importance of the father in the case, and of his patient's role as a daughter. He notices that her father constantly accompanies Miss K to the hospital and even to the treatment room while she often speaks of writing to her father. Miss K's relationship with her father inevitably involves the mother also, and the mother's relationship with her husband and her daughter. Thus the therapist becomes aware in treating Miss K of the importance of her father and mother as we have illustrated in Fig. 10a, and that this disturbance involves the mutual relationship of all three.

The classical method for dealing with such a triangular relationship is ideally for each of the individuals involved to see separate therapists. The daughter sees a therapist (No. 1), the father sees a therapist (No. 2), and the mother sees a therapist (No. 3), as illustrated in Fig. 10b. In each of these individual situations it would be obvious to the therapist concerned that the other parties in the triangular situation were closely involved, but

Fig. 9

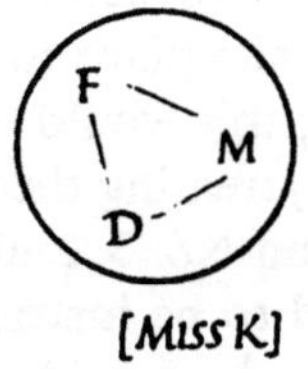

D [Miss K] = P [Miss K]

Fig. 10

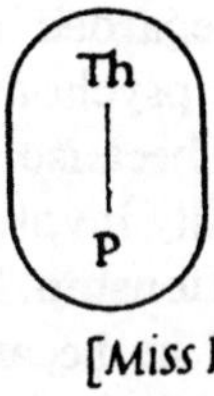

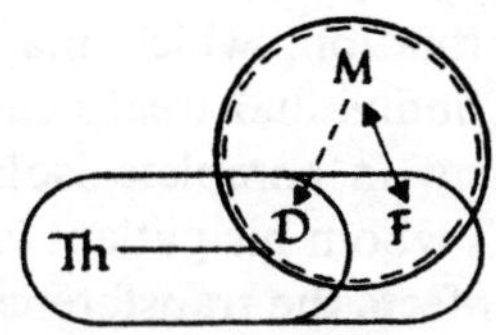

Fig. 10a

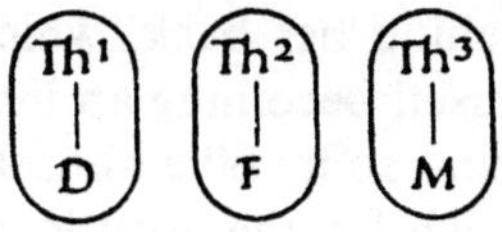

Fig. 10b

Fig. 11

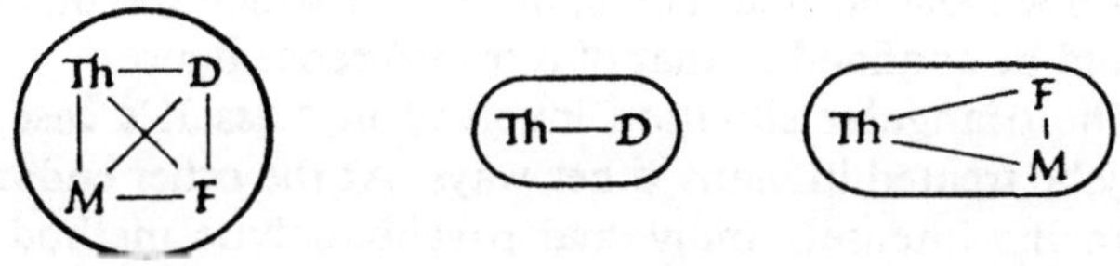

Fig. 12

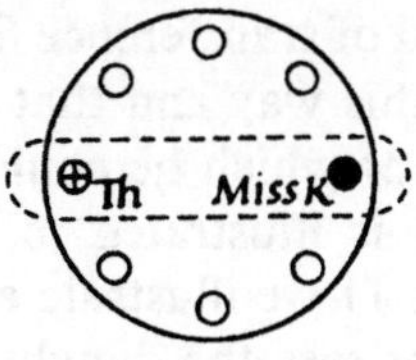

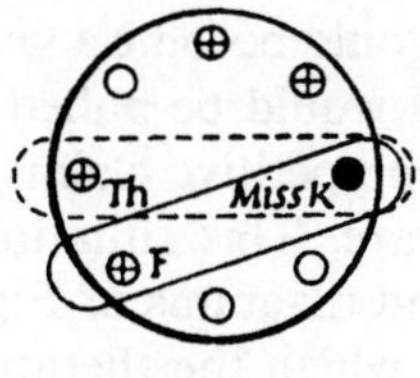

Fig. 12a

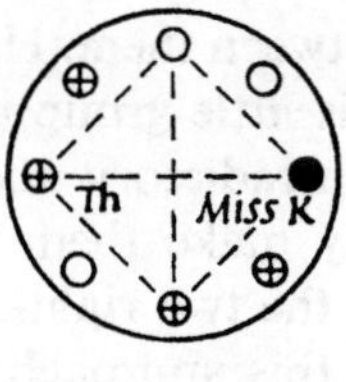

Fig. 12b

he would have no contact with the other two people nor with their therapists, so that treatment would take place in three isolated therapeutic fields. In psychoanalysis, this would literally be the pattern of treatment and analyst No. 1, treating the daughter, would prefer not to meet analysts No. 2 and No. 3, and certainly not the father or mother. If he felt bound to be instrumental in arranging treatment for father and mother, he would see neither of them himself and would send each of them to different analysts.

There are very good reasons for such a procedure in the strict psychoanalytic situation, which may be regarded as the most extreme form of individual treatment. The psychoanalyst needs to treat his patient in complete isolation, because to meet the other people with whom his patient is actually involved, disturbs and, as it were, infects the transference relationship. The psychoanalyst would feel in Miss K's case that if he became involved with her father and mother he would soon find himself talking about Miss K behind her back, which would be distasteful; or he might find himself becoming an intermediary between Miss K and her parents and so involve himself hopelessly in a triangular conflict, from which for therapeutic reasons he needs to remain detached. Fig. 10b illustrates the pattern which a psychoanalytic treatment of the triangular situation would produce. There would be three isolated treatments, in each of which the therapist's role would be confined to that of a transference figure.

The triangular situation involved in Miss K's case, however, may be treated in many other ways. At the other end of the scale from the intensely individual psychoanalytic method would be that of a group analyst who saw father, mother, and daughter together. By doing this he would participate in the real situation and would be able to observe directly the various roles assigned to him by the patients and the significance of the interactions between them. He would become a kind of transference figure for this little group and would be pulled this way and that by their contradictory and competitive claims, of which he could gradually make them aware. This situation is illustrated in Fig. 11. In the two right-hand diagrams of Fig. 11 we illustrate a variant of this approach in which the therapist sees the daughter alone and sees the father and mother together.

We can see therefore that the original triangular situation which became manifest in Miss K's case can be treated either by isolated individual therapy as in Fig. 10b or in a group, in this case a family group as illustrated in Fig. 11. It could also be treated in one of the therapeutic groups we have described, and we shall now examine how Miss K's conflict will pattern itself against this background.

In a therapeutic group among six or seven total strangers we would expect Miss K to manifest her conflict, but with a certain difference. The very strong need which she felt to monopolize her father in the family situation would probably appear now as a need to monopolize the therapist, and if her need was too strong for her to tolerate the group he might gratify it by taking her out of the group into individual treatment. Whether or not the therapist decided to do this, Miss K would have replaced her feelings for her real father by a transference relationship in the group as illustrated in Fig. 12, and this could be analysed. This transference pattern might take a different form if Miss K happened to transfer her feelings for her father on to another patient (Fig. 12a), or it might be further elaborated in a mixed group by the transference of her feelings for her mother on to a female patient at the same time (Fig. 12b). If Miss K re-established the whole triangular situation in terms of transference within the group the pattern of the situation becomes very similar to that illustrated in Fig. 11 but with the salient difference that this situation is now recreated in terms of transference and that the remaining members of the group are also present. They may act simply as a background for the drama, or they may be called on to represent people outside Miss K's immediate family circle, or to witness events, or to take sides, or to act as auxiliaries to the therapist.

Perhaps we can now see more clearly how these various patterns of treatment relate to one another and to the original situation. The original situation presents a conflict involving daughter, father, and mother, which ideally requires that all three should be treated. In Fig. 10 we see how the conflict is treated in three isolated situations (as in pure psychoanalysis), in each of which the original situation will appear as a background.

In Fig. 11 we see the family of three treated as a group ('root'-group). The approach is made from quite a different angle and opens up the possibility of group treatment as a pattern of treatment in its own right. It is in many ways the exact opposite of the treatment situation shown in Fig. 10 from which all relationships except the transference relationship to the therapist are excluded. The modification of the transference relationship raises many technical problems to offset other advantages but we must forego a discussion of these here.

The situation in Fig. 12 shows a transference relationship, this time in a group-analytic group, in which the individual members react not only as individuals but as interrelated members of a group situation integrating the behaviour of all. Her personal need to monopolize the therapist in a father role clearly appears, and she may also transfer her feelings for her mother to another member, as in Fig. 12b. What is not seen so readily from the diagram is that the mother role, for example, may be transferred on to the group as a whole rather than on to any one individual member. Here we see the original family pattern re-established through transferences in terms of group relationships and at this point we may be surprised to note that the essentials of the therapeutic situations illustrated in Figs. 10 and 11 are now combined. The situation in Fig. 11 is re-established by virtue of the fact that all members of the original triangle are present, as far as Miss K is concerned, through the creation of transference relationship within the group ('T'-group). At the same time the conditions of Fig. 10 are present because Miss K is again the only member of her family in treatment with the therapist and because the development of a full transference situation is now possible and there is nothing to prevent the therapist from acting in a purely therapeutic capacity. There is no need for him to take sides or to become involved as a person in the family conflict and so compromise his position as a therapist.

An example of a critical period in a group. The following report should help to make more concrete what is meant by the group situation as a whole, as a matrix of all individual processes. For professional reasons this illustration is in the most general terms.

In this group in which things proceed rapidly and intensively there are signs of increasing tension. These signs could appear to call for a purely individual interpretation. Two members were recently involved in serious tragedies concerning very close relations outside. Another went through a very serious illness which could only be dealt with by an operation. Others had special circumstances to blame for missing sessions, and one left the group altogether. Apart from the multiplication of events there are many indications that these apparently isolated incidents are connected with the goings-on inside the group itself. The group understands this well enough. Further signs of unresolved tension accumulate. Two patients – again without knowing of each other – asked to be seen privately, alone. They revealed matters which to them are serious ones indeed and charged with deep emotion. One of them stated that he would not trust himself at this stage to speak about these concerns to the group.

In the session itself hesitations to speak out are manifest and admitted. Someone will say 'I will undoubtedly make my contribution, but at the moment I am trembling to think of it, and cannot yet trust. . . .' Under increasing inner pressure some members now begin to make such contributions of a more personal nature. It becomes more and more clear that whereas each individual member had his or her own reasons for hesitating, *there is something in the total situation*, some difficulty, some barrier, which the group has in common, each has it with the others, each has it with the group. This was also pointed out, and is an example of an interpretation which concerns the group rather than individuals. One member observed that gradually people have actually said much more, but always under provocation; they have to be provoked, but do not feel at ease to come forward spontaneously. Someone else remarked, quite rightly, that it seems that almost all, if not all, of the group members had incestuous complications in their lives. This does not mean that any of these patients actually committed incest. What was meant is that members had intimate relationships which, in a transference sense, were too close to their infantile (parental) objects.

At this stage the conductor pointed out that this very same thing seemed to be reflected in seeking individual interviews, with their professional secrecy, their opportunity for confidential confession, and also in the fear of the group (community) and the mistrust of others. It was now for the group to see how they could deal with these problems, or to acknowledge, if this is the case, that they cannot do so.

Various interesting points are illustrated in this report. Deep 'oedipal' conflicts – which psychoanalysis has revealed to be of central importance in the genesis of psychoneurotic and allied pathological mental conditions – are here laid bare. These are most certainly operative in each of the individuals concerned. If these conflicts are operating in strength and depth the elaborate day-by-day working through of individual psychoanalysis may be called for. It must be mentioned, however, that most of these particular patients have undergone more or less lengthy periods of psychoanalytical treatment in the past.

In line with the fact that this same oedipal conflict is a universal heritage of mankind in childhood, it appears here also as a common background of the group. In the immediate context of this group individual, personal suffering and symptoms are manifest and conscious, but the common ground of defensive reaction in the group is not. The way in which it eventually becomes evident to the group reveals at the same time some technical detail, and illustrates the nature of a 'group-centred' type of interpretation. The way in which the members of this group actively participate in the analytic process is also illuminated. Mention may also be made of the signs of increasing tension in their variety, as well as its resolution.

The successful analysis of the meaning of the call for individual interview, both in the immediately presenting ('here-and-now') situation *and* in its deeper significance as well as its additional transference character, deserves to be pointed out once more.

For further clinical material the reader is referred to the account of children's and adolescents' groups in Chapter 8. In their way, adult groups are as dramatic, expressive, and meaningful as these children's groups are, but naturally of greater complexity; there is the additional difficulty of giving material fully without violating discretion. Essentially the principles of group-analytic psychotherapy hold good in any therapeutic situation, allowing for flexible modifications to suit the actual circumstances.

When working with children, especially with younger ones, there is more emphasis on activity. In group-analytic terms the group members have an *occupation.* Nevertheless recent developments have interestingly enough led to an approximation to the group-analytic approach to adults, with slightly greater emphasis on verbal expression, where the aim of treatment is a more radical one.

The illustrations given of children's groups clearly bring out the operation of such dynamic concepts as the group as a whole, dramatization, and the location of a disturbance as part of a figurational analysis.

The institutional setting described with its interlocking groups is an excellent example of the application of the group-analytic method operating in a circumscribed community.* With this example (pp. 227–30) we can once more throw light on our concept of the multipersonal network of mental conflict. Treating only the individual patient without giving attention to his network is not enough. Both the network of family ties at home, and the current network of doctors, nurses, teachers, and other staff are considered important. In a child this is even easier to see and treat than it is in an adult, who will bring into the treatment situation also his now internalized conflicts dating back to his own childhood. In the current treatment situation these will show as transference reactions in so far as the individual patient by himself is concerned.

The observations made regarding groups of prepubertal boys and girls are of particular interest. The therapeutic experience is a 'demasculinizing demand on the active, aggressive boy, required to be resisted to the end. Surrender in the girl's group signified the emergence of active, angry, envious wishes . . .' (see page 215).

Such observations made about these groups of boys and girls confirm Freud's conclusion that the most fundamental fear in men is of sexual passivity to another man, and that the most fundamental fear in women is the absence of an active male organ, which is interpreted as castration ('penis envy').

* Compare this also with accounts of the community at Northfield Military Neurosis Centre, e.g. in S. H. Foulkes: *Therapeutic Group Analysis*, and page 239 below.

Chapter 6

The Natural History of the Therapeutic Group

The psychotherapeutic group is a mirror not only for the patient but also for the analytic theorist, who can look in on this complex scene and note what he will. There are no limits to the possible descriptive subtleties open to him, and he may find himself exhibiting surprisingly different group models from those of his colleagues. Conceptions will alter with preconceptions. Certain aspects of these conceptual models, however, tend to repeat themselves.

The living portrait of the group is most uniformly painted in terms of conflict, which is evident in manifest or latent forms in every group situation. It may be conflict brought in by an individual, or conflict arising autochthonously from the matrix of the group and its developments. There is, for example, ample provocation in the setting itself to set going a life-long defiance. The freedom of the group situation may unleash the monopolist or exhibitionist and leave the rebel with nothing to rebel against save time and space. He may respond with open irritability and hostility, or by an exaggerated show of boredom. His problem is learning to live with his group neighbours in the limited 'living space' of the group, and accommodating himself to their 'elbowing'.

In the early stages of a group's life (and in very inhibited groups) there may be much anxiety and guilt in individual members over their time consumption. At times they may seem almost to line up, problems in hand, with the infinite docility of a bus queue. Longer group experience brings more peremptory attitudes and diminution in social restraint.

1. SOME OBSERVATIONS ON HUMAN CONFLICT

Conflict is so pervasive in the therapeutic situation that to specify any particular manifestation of it, however helpful to exposition, introduces distinctions that are wholly artificial and out of context.

With this proviso in mind, we will deal in turn with the conflicts over conformity, authority, dependency, and change, all of which may at some time or other become burning questions for the group. They present different aspects of an overall conflict over dominance in the basic sense of the parent's dominance over the child. It is the primary conflict of man as a group animal.

The individual in any group must behave himself according to the standards imposed by the group. These standards approximate to the average behaviour of the individual members. Individuals may deviate to a larger or smaller extent from a hypothetical (statistical) 'norm' and the degree of deviation determines the 'individuality' of the individual. The inner pressures at work drive him either to excessive conformity with the 'norm' or to cultivation and exaggeration of his 'individuality'.

To what extent he does the one or the other is partly a matter of his cultural milieu (meaning by this, the socially relevant environment as a whole) and partly a question of the inherited 'constitution' and upbringing which help to make up his personality. In primitive cultures, where there is greater homogeneity of social institutions and more resemblance in the basic personality structure, individuals tend towards exaggerated conformity, whereas in certain parts of the western world there appears to be a premium on 'rugged individualism' and 'cut-throat competition'.

But however homogeneous the culture, and however extensive and intensive the treatment is in even the most conforming, the narcissistic, egocentric core persists, and struggles to persist against every environmental threat of submersion. We can only experience reality in ourselves, and even the most primitive must recognize the self within them. As William James* put it: 'The axis of reality runs solely through the egoistic places – they are strung upon it like so many beads.' The self is always the ultimate reference, and environment meets the self somewhere *inside* the self. Although one may talk loosely of the 'group ego', there is nothing analogous with self-feeling in the group outside the individual. In all states of group cohesion, the self remains (to quote James again) 'the storm centre, the origin of co-ordinates, the constant place of stress'.

The second conflict theme concerns reactions to authority and authority figures. The individual brings his authoritarian problem

* In *The Principles of Psychology.*

– his 'father complex' – into the centre of events from the very beginning, and directs it with full force at the therapist. During the early stages it often assumes the guise of petty quibbling over the group 'rules' or constant late attendances which are excused with a bland air. Feelings for the therapist (as for the father) are not unmixed. The ambivalence may take subtle forms of expression but the good feelings are always counterbalanced by hostility (sarcasm, mocking, teasing). Open hostility is seldom possible because of the deep inner fears that centred round the father originally.

In one group a patient of this type sat through many group meetings displacing most of this 'father' aggression on to the members of the group, leaving the therapist conspicuously alone. One day, after a protracted silence, he was highly stimulated by the defiance of another patient (who had made use of a 'dirty' expression), and bending down by the fireplace he extracted a lump of coal and put it on the central table in the full view of the group, at the same time remarking with great satisfaction: 'That's something I have wanted to do for a long time.' He then stared rebelliously at the therapist awaiting his reaction. When nothing was said or done, he took up the coal and put it back in the fireplace.

This symbolic defiance on an infantile plane is a striking example of the difficulties these patients have in manipulating their aggressive drives successfully and satisfactorily. It is also a good example of 'acting out' in the group situation, a form of symptomatic behaviour that can be used for a therapeutic end. 'Acting out' in this way outside the therapeutic situation is a form of resistance to treatment and should be discouraged.

The third conflict theme revolves round the problem of dependency. Group development is in many respects analogous to child development. The conflicts over dependency are crucial ones for both situations, and their normal resolution is a matter of wise management on the part of therapist and parent.

The therapist's attitude is, in essence, a reluctance to accept an authoritarian role and a preference for working through and with the group with as little interference as possible. The conductor's aim is to wean the group from its leader-centredness.

The contemporary attitude in child training and education is not dissimilar. The drift is from scheduled to self-demanding need satisfactions. The child rears itself under the guidance of the parent, and educates itself under the guidance of its teachers. In functional education, the child is not taught, but given every opportunity to teach himself.

The same is true of group-analysis. The analyst offers his patients every opportunity and encouragement in the group-analytic situation to cure themselves – and each other. The therapeutic process could not take place without his specific contribution, however.

The child is expected to mature beyond his childish belief in the omnipotent parent. He must learn to stand on his own two feet and dig in his own ten toes when the need arises. He should not, eventually, wish to dominate or be dominated, crawl before authority, or remain everlastingly resentful and rebellious towards it.

If this unfortunate state ensues, he will be fated to carry the unhappy 'complex' into every subsequent group situation in life. When, at last, he reaches a psychotherapeutic group, he will pass through stages of bewilderment and resentment because the analyst fails to live up to his authoritarian expectations. If and when he begins to understand the conductor's role in the group, he is on his way to recovery.

Kurt Lewin, in a series of brilliant studies on authoritarian versus democratic regimes, showed fairly conclusively that authoritarian group 'climates' create authoritarian personalities and democratic groups breed democrats. It is for the same good reasons that group-analytic psychotherapy has been called a training for democracy, meaning by that the inculcation of an outlook happily adjusted to all aspects of its environment and making no undue demands upon it.

The form that the dependency conflict takes in life varies with the age of the individual. It lies behind other developmental events and is coloured by them. The intra-uterine dependency becomes the breast dependency, which becomes the parent dependency and so on, until adolescence is reached, when the classical crisis takes place. Adolescent dependency is a conflict waged in more mature terms – finance, living out, boy friends, late nights, supervision, etc. Although engaged in regressive struggles, the perspective of the adolescent is towards the future and he is preoccupied with his progression towards it.

In the psychotherapeutic group, it is more this picture of the dependency theme that is seen, but it should be understood that all such seemingly adult conflicts are reactivations of infantile ones.

A young housewife had been a 'model child' (a term full of disastrous meanings to the child psychiatrist) and extremely dependent on her mother. Being an only child, this dependency was fostered. As in all such cases, there was strong resentment and hostility which was quite unable to obtain expression in view of the 'goodness' of the mother and her unfailing kindness and helpfulness. In time the child became a young girl and the girl a young woman; and the young woman got herself married. She now had a double prop, but also a very distressing symptom, which made it almost impossible for her to be left alone under certain circumstances. After a year's analysis of this situation in the group, she reported that things were becoming intolerable at home, and life with mother was now a constant struggle. She tried to transfer her dependency on to the therapist, and when this failed, she became considerably distressed and contemplated leaving the group. She was openly aggressive towards her mother and made plans to find a new home. (She was still living with her husband in her mother's house and occupying the bedroom of her childhood.) 'And on top of all this,' she complained, 'my husband's as pleased as punch, because he says that I'm at last standing on my own feet.' But if this was to be the outcome of group treatment, she did not like it at all. However, she remained on in the group, and the story is still unended.

We come now to the last of our conflicts (but by no means the last of the group's conflicts) – the conflict over change. It is a common fear in the patient coming to psychotherapy that therapeutic change will imply the loss of a precious idiosyncrasy and the 'ironing out' of a not unprepossessing 'ego'. The more narcissistic the patient, the more apparent is this fear. As one patient remarked; 'I know I suffer a great deal through being so highly sensitive, but I don't want the treatment to change that, because then it wouldn't be me.' This apprehension, however, is based on a misconception of the therapeutic purpose, which is to cure neurosis and not uproot important sublimations. In the psychotherapeutic group, the sound part of the individuality is given firm roots. The group respects its development and free emergence, but is rightly intolerant of false claims and distorted self-assessments. The group process, whilst reinforcing the shared basic structures, loosens neurotic inhibitions, and allows a freer development of individual differences.

One of the basic resistances of the patient and of the group is the resistance to change – change either in themselves or in their environment.

In a group made up entirely of young married women, someone raised the topic of winning a large sum of money on the football pools. All seven without exception declined to have anything to do at all with such a windfall. 'It only brings trouble and misery; people sponge on you and hate you; one chap died soon after a win; it makes you get snobbish and disliked; I would much rather have things as they are.' . . . As they are! neurosis and all; unhappy marriages, dilapidated houses, money troubles . . . but no change. And why? One of them said: 'Because if you didn't have all those things, something dreadful else might happen.' The unhappy lot was a security against an even unhappier lot. Change was the great unknown. It was always the case of 'better the devil you know', even if that devil used mental torture and lived inside you. The inner dilapidations were also a safeguard against the insatiable demands of conscience which made cowards of them all.

But change is implicit in all treatment. Does the patient's coming to treatment signify a desire for change? One must remember, as George Bach points out, that 'the patient's wish for help and health is ambivalent'. Under it lie 'neurotically distorted wishes' which have nothing to do with treatment and getting better. He apparently comes to be cured, but actually he comes not to be changed but to be approved of. All his resistances (and they sum up with other resistances into group resistances) are directed towards maintaining the *status quo*. And if he can keep the group from changing, there will be further self-protection. He will therefore resist all group changes – new members coming in and old members leaving, changing of seats and changing of times, and above all, any group developments into new and unfamiliar psychological territory. At the crucial point he will oppose all analytic interpretations either from the group or from the therapist.

A point of some importance to both patient and therapist is the observable sign (or signs) of changes, and by change here is implied change for the better.

The layman is inclined, from analogy with the physical illness, to look for the more concrete manifestations of improvement. The cinema may have been his mentor in the matter. The dreary housewife of the first reel, weighed down with depression and inferiority, is emancipated by treatment in a spectacular fashion and emerges, in the finale, as a carefree, well-dressed, and self-assured woman, obviously years younger than her former self and many times as attractive. This large outward change is taken to be a reflection of an equally large internal rehabilitation.

The therapist might well be suspicious of the 'painted smile', and see in it nothing more than a defence against actual inner change. He will wisely put his trust in the small 'dynamic shifts' – the little jolt from the coupling engine that transmits itself throughout the train – of such gradual occurrence that when eventually brought to the notice of the patient himself, he sees in it only something 'obvious', and can hardly believe that it has not always been so. (It was not without reason that Freud referred to psychoanalysis as the psychology of the obvious.)

The therapist will therefore be more content with small inner changes than large outer ones, and he will hope for many therapeutic repercussions to set in, reaching out in time and combining to bring about changes long after the treatment is concluded. The external treatment may have come to an end, but the internal therapeutic process will go on.

This attitude to change is best summed up in some lines from William James: 'I am done with great things and big things, great institutions and big success, and I am for those tiny, invisible, molecular, moral forces that work from individual to individual, creeping through the crannies of the world like so many soft rootlets, or like capillary oozing of water, yet which, if given time, will rend the hardest monuments of man's pride.'

What harder monument of man's pride is there than his neurosis?

2. SOME HYPOTHETICAL STAGES

It might have been thought that these various conflict themes would have provided some basis for an evolutionary classification, but this has not proved to be the case. Group-analytic psychotherapy has come to regard the clear-cut stages given by some authors as procrustean beds into which the group is willy-nilly fitted. It accepts the conflict themes and their temporal developments in the group in the form of manifest and latent movements, but it protests at stratifying the processes.

Others have been less hesitant in this respect. One classificatory method has been through theme analysis. From an analysis of many group protocols, it was found (Powdermaker and Frank, 1953) that certain themes recurred with exceptional frequency:

(*a*) Mixed feelings towards loving women.
(*b*) Hostility, distrust, and fear of people.
(*c*) Feelings of inferiority and desires to be average.
(*d*) The problem of blaming others or accepting the responsibility of our own actions.

These topics would catch and hold the interest of the group for longer periods than any other, but even they underwent a characteristic cycle. Out of a silence would come one of these topics; gradually the whole group would become involved in an interchange, possibly a 'chain' reaction (see Chapter 7); and finally there would be a gradual waxing of interest until a point of 'theme satiation' is reached.

George Bach* has developed an elaborate system of group development. Seven phases of group development subsume seven levels of communication, seven different types of resistance, and seven therapeutic functions. Running through the phases there are sixteen characteristic themes.

During the first phase, the members 'test out' the group situation so as to make themselves familiar with its possibilities and limitations. They then look to the conductor and centre all their therapeutic hopes on him. The next three phases are somewhat 'stormy' and emotionally intense. They begin by going back in time to the playing out of their family roles and vying with each other in their thematic productions. The role-playing gradually becomes more and more fanciful and there is a great deal of associated affective discharge. In the last two stages, they take a more serious view of themselves as a group, and interest themselves in its structure and function. The seventh pillar of wisdom enables them to engage in deep analytic interpretations, in contrast to the superficial giving and taking of advice characteristic of earlier phases. Bach suggests that Bion's (see Chapter 1) 'basic assumptions' and 'work' groups might well fit in with his own developmental scheme, if one could imagine the 'assumptions' evolving steadily from dependency, through pairing and fighting and fleeing, to work.

* G. R. Bach, *Intensive Group Psychotherapy* Ronald, Press, New York, 1954.

The patients in Bach's analytic groups begin their group life by talking of the problems that have brought them into treatment, and what they hope from coming. New patients tend to give 'confessional' material as part of the initiation ordeal. They go on to talk in broad intellectual terms about techniques, theories, aims, and objects, but break off to blame the environment in all its shapes and forms for their miseries. Then comes a period when they discuss their past in terms of childhood incidents and family relationships. At this point they begin the frustrating business of giving but not taking advice, and, in fact, acting resentfully to advice that is given. Dream reporting may occur from the second phase onwards, but the group improves in its interpretative capacity as time goes on. By this time, they are fully conscious of the group as such and show an awareness of group atmospheres. The discussion centres on group themes such as role-playing, the functions of the conductor, etc. They develop very much into an in-group (topological term) and separate what happens within the group carefully from outside living. They interest themselves in latecomers and absentees, the problems of the isolated ones, the ones that pair off, and the sub-groups. They express their feelings for each other and discuss them openly and analytically. They show great interest in the opinions of the others about them.

These lists, of course, do not by any means exhaust the topics that interest a group. Allowing for a great deal of elasticity they do show a slight tendency to evolve in some order, but not, we think, with such detailed consistency. Bach's list can be examined as an illustration of the possibilities, but his classificatory zeal frequently gets the better of him. He has also a list of values (14 of them derived from the Murray–Allport list) which he tries to fit into his developmental scheme. These include such 'values' as health, property, authority, sex, prestige, leadership, physical attractiveness, friendships, and so on, omitting some couched in Murray's barbarous terminology. According to Bach, sex lies low during all but two phases, when it becomes an acute topic; these are the middle phases of four and five, when group life is altogether disturbed.

A. Wolf has not only envisaged stages but sets his group the task of moving along in accordance with them. This programmatic method may be expected to tell us something about its value as a therapeutic procedure, but possibly less about group dynamics, for which spontaneity in development is a prerequisite.

Given a free and flexible group situation, without tests, questionnaires, or drawings, with the accent on verbal communications in the form of 'free-floating' discussion, what is likely to happen? The immediate answer is 'anything'. But we must take this a little further.

Every group must have at least a beginning and an end (even when the group dies of 'exhaustion', to use Freud's expression). Somewhere between the initial and final periods (for periods they are, and not moments in time) must lie an intermediate phase.

Now it may be true to say that every group begins differently, develops differently, and ends differently, but are they not all group-analytic groups of seven or eight patients looking at each other from the margins of a small circle? And may we not expect, then, some family resemblances, keeping in mind, all the while, that our stages are as variable as our groups, and every session is different from every other? Having stated all this, we can now, cautiously, look for similarities.

The initial phase. Bach has called this, with some justification, the period of the 'therapeutic honeymoon'. It is the stage of magical thinking projected on to the therapist. He becomes the One-who-knows or the One-who-cures, and expectations of a rapid recovery are high. When these hopes are dashed, the patient may derive a great deal of incidental satisfaction and benefit from his acceptance by the therapist and the group. He may make this group support the final expression of his treatment and will repudiate the function of analysis when it begins.

The initiation into a group can be considerably softened by the therapist's gentle management of introductions and his own calm acceptance of the situation, strange though it may seem to be.

The patients, feeling a little self-conscious and nervous, may wait expectantly for some instruction or direction. They may ask the therapist directly for guidance on procedure, and may be rather taken aback when they are told in reply to talk about anything that they want to or that comes into their minds. Well, a great deal enters their heads in this unusual situation – they may, for instance, find the man's drooping moustache across the circle very funny, but it would be, they think, decidedly rude to mention such a thing. They begin to wonder what the therapist would say if they talked about cricket or gardening. They may ask him just this, and receive a non-committal response. *If* that is what they feel they have come all the way from North London, heavy with anxiety, to talk about, they must go ahead. This returns them to the subject of their problems and symptoms over which they have brooded for months or even years. When you attend a doctor with a physical illness, your immediate impulse is not to talk about cricket or gardening but about your painful symptoms. Your feelings about them, however, are fairly straightforward. You want to be rid of them as soon as possible. There is no reluctance to tell, and no difficulty about telling, unless you have some special speech impediment. The psychological symptom, on the other hand, is felt to be less 'respectable'. It has something to do, the patient thinks, with inferiority or weakness. He has nothing to show for it, as he would have in the case of a physical ailment, and he discovers from experience that people as a rule feel less sorry for him because they hold the same opinion of the symptom as he does himself. He may have already endured with diminishing fortitude 'pep' talks ranging from 'pull yourself together' to 'you think too much about yourself; it's just imagination, pure and simple'. It *is* imagination, but a deep and inaccessible part of it is in the realm of unconscious phantasy, which is never pure and simple. The language for describing these strange inner feelings – the feelings of not being yourself, of feeling different, or of being overwhelmed by some unknown fear (unknown because it is unconscious) that seems to paralyse your mind and body, feelings of madness and badness and sadness in a confusing mixture and served up with guilt and apprehension – the language for putting these into adequate words has yet to be invented. This is responsible for the despairing sense of being 'cut off' from people, of being unable to 'get across' any of the fears that trouble. And who has the patience or tolerance to listen whilst you mumble and moan about incommunicable things?

Here we have the basic problem of communication again. The neurotic patient must learn how to formulate in words his ineluctable experiences, and to find someone to listen to him. When the infant is learning to speak, he passes through stages of babbling and jargon, and for a long time finds it difficult to express himself adequately. In his environment, however, he is fortunate in having a set of people whose business in life seems to be to listen patiently and helpfully to him. Twenty years later, when he starts to learn a foreign language, he will experience it all over again, but with a difference. He has now to pay people to listen to him helpfully and patiently. Everyone else is highly intolerant. The language of neurosis is a private one, belonging, with its signs and symbols, to the age of infancy when symptoms are made. This infantile language needs to be translated into adult speech before it can be understood. It is one of the group's functions to assist in this translation. The wordless feelings have to be worded. The group-analytic situation has been created to listen, patiently and helpfully, for these first words, and to encourage the patient to extend his range of communication. To understand is to begin to cure.

The therapist is, therefore, fairly confident that when the patients begin to talk, they will either talk about what matters to them, or defend themselves against talking about it; but sooner or later, they will return to it because they cannot get away from it. He can leave it to them and wait.

In this initial period it is natural for the patients to turn to the therapist and address him personally. This is founded on their life-long experience and expectation of the doctor–patient relationship. It also seems sensible to them to conduct their treatment in the form of question and answer. They ask the 'expert' and he gives them an answer. But not in the group-analytic situation. To their surprise (and the situation is full of surprises of this nature) he returns them their question or poses a counter-question. A question cannot be answered by a question, but the second question may set going a new train of thought that may reach out to the answer. The therapist may also, and is more likely to, throw the question open to the group.

This brings the patient for the first time up against the group. He must re-orient himself away from the doctor-to-patient axis, and towards the patient-to-patient axis. He is incredulous at first at being 'treated' by a 'fellow mortal'. But if a group of them are competent to judge you and hang you when you err, then a group of them (selected with much greater care) should be credited with some capacity at least – with a therapist in attendance – to assess your difficulties and cure them.

Very soon, the patients in the group get down to discussing their individual symptoms and here they find that they have so many in common that the pressing sense of isolation begins to lift.

Each member is preoccupied with 'me' and tries his best to put this essential 'me' before the group. Of course, he decks it up a bit for the occasion, and emphasizes that although 'me' suffers from these many symptoms (*a*) it is not its fault at all, and (*b*) it is really a very nice 'me' at heart.

The others in the group still remain strangers, and seem strange and different. At this stage, newcomers are accepted without much fuss, and members may leave with little comment. Symptom discussions predominate, but even the longest list of symptoms must come to an end at some time; and then there is silence, and silences in the early days can be embarrassing. Nervous movements begin to show themselves in a manner fairly characteristic for the individual. Some may cross and uncross their legs, some may pick at their fingers, some may rotate their rings, and some may twist their handkerchiefs. Eyes are accommodated neutrally to the floor or to the distance. Each one feels exposed and vulnerable, and hopes desperately that some bold spirit will break into the silence and set life going again. The silences seem to have the timelessness of eternity about them.

The group look to the therapist to give them a lead, but he seems to be waiting as well, but without anxiety. They wonder what he is waiting for. What does he expect from them? They feel quite certain that they are not doing what he hopes they will do. But what can it be? He doesn't say.

Someone begins to talk at last, and there is a general sigh of relief. But if this is going to happen every time, it will be a strain. Last session, they had to have an aspirin when they got home.

Husband asked: 'What do you do?' ... 'Impossible to explain. ... We talk.' ... 'About what?' ... 'About anything. Everything. ... I don't know. We just talk.' ... 'And what does the doctor do?' ... 'Nothing. Oh, he just talks as well. Much less than we do, though. He doesn't seem to say much at all. Perhaps he's only a beginner.'

The real beginner, of course, is the patient, and he has still a lot to learn – about groups, and about himself. But this is the stage of perplexity, of getting to know what it is all about, and who's who, and what's wrong with them.

The tensions of initiation pass, and the group begins to settle down. Sometimes there is a 'confessional' stage, with some relief from anxiety and guilt. The 'secrets' seem much less noxious when revealed.

They find pleasure now in meeting each other once a week, and may even look forward to it. They remember things to tell the group. They do not as yet have group dreams.

The intermediate phase. Almost everything in this book may be said to happen during this stage, but we will attempt to simplify the picture for the record.

The group now truly becomes a group. Their centre of reference is no longer the therapist alone, but they remain as conscious of his presence in the group, even when he is quite silent. They are aware that he is always listening to them, and at certain frustrated moments they may accuse him roundly of knowing the answers and yet withholding them. He becomes sadistic and cruel, or human and helpful, depending on their own moods. Their perceptions are very much determined by their feelings and the state of what has been called their 'assumptive worlds' (Abercrombie).

They address each other and respond directly to each other. They form sub-groups within the group, and try to meet outside. They keep 'secrets' from the therapist, and declare that they talk much more freely in his absence. They wonder that he never gets ill. They are vitally interested in what goes on in the group, although at times they complain of intense boredom. They investigate each other's histories. Occasionally they may become very angry with one another, but they can say so, and it doesn't seem to matter so much. They find out what their anger means and what its antecedents are.

Sometimes their symptoms are relieved by a session, but often they are made worse, and they begin to wonder whether the symptom really wants to get cured, and whether it may not be in two minds about it. The symptom's reaction to the group seems to depend on the group's reaction to the symptom, and whether they neglect it or cosset it.

With the stage of support, mutually enjoyed, comes the analysis, and the deeper this is the more resistance it meets. The group start to interpret their own interactions and to uncover their hostile and sexual feelings. They become therapists gradually, and almost in spite of themselves; and they are not fully aware what good therapists they are or even that they are being therapeutic at all.

If this phase is allowed to go on for too long, the members may become 'group addicted' and feel that they cannot carry on without the help of the group. They are as dependent on the group now as they previously were on the therapist. The new problem is to wean them from the group.

The group at this 'interminable' stage is an 'encapsulated society'. They resent newcomers and may combine to drive them away. They equally resent anyone leaving the group and may struggle for his retention. Their state is one of stalemate, and they seem to move neither backwards nor forwards. Their topics show a tendency to circularity, and they frustrate themselves with their own repetitiousness.

Before this point has been reached, the wise therapist has introduced the group to the idea of its impending dissolution, or perhaps reshuffled it and brought in 'fresh blood' from outside.

The terminal phase. Termination of any therapeutic situation should always be gradual, to allow the patient a chance to 'work through' the many anxieties and depressions that, in therapy as in life, associate themselves with endings. Endings seem to lead to reflections on the futility of life and the inevitability of death.

Some analysts prefer to set a time limit beforehand to a group, but it must be remembered that this prior knowledge is likely to affect their behaviour at all stages. The end in these cases is always in view, but, like the image of death, is repressed. Resistances peculiar to this special knowledge make their appearance. Some members may find this therapeutic pressure difficult to bear.

Another method of termination is to hold an anniversary review every year so that the group can make themselves familiar with the idea and keep it somewhere in mind even if out of sight.

When confronted with the end, the group invariably finds many good and logical reasons for continuing, and these must be carefully analysed. They may resuscitate some of their forgotten symptoms or produce a few new ones. Their earlier dependency on the conductor may reaffirm itself as a transient phenomenon.

The conductor is, himself, a little more active than he was during the intermediate stage, and his activity is directed towards returning his patients back to normal life without any props. This presents fewer difficulties than in the individual therapeutic situation, which is more divorced from life. The great advantage of group-analysis is realized precisely at this point. It occupies a position midway between the autistic, unreal world of the individual psychotherapeutic situation and the very real social situations in the world outside the clinic. The transition is therefore smoother, and readjustment to reality and its demands easier. 'Life outside' is not so different from the 'miniature society' of group-analysis, and in spirit at least, every group is an open one – open to the 'free ocean of life' outside.

3. A LITERARY EXAMPLE OF A CLOSED GROUP

By not admitting or discharging members, the closed group creates a peculiar intensity of its own, a brilliant phantasy example of which occurs in Sartre's *In Camera*. The readers will well remember that room in Hell where the small group of three collects. It is a room without mirrors in which the members are forced to see themselves and are unable to close their eyes to each other for their eyelids have disappeared – *Il faut vivre les yeux ouverts . . . pour toujours* – they read their judgements in one another's eyes. Not only have their eyelids disappeared, but the session is an interminable one, and the doors are apparently closed. In addition to the three members, there is another character, the valet, who belongs to the situation, who makes the introductions and who is there to answer the initial questions, but who for the most part allows the members to interact with each other. He is there to serve the group, if they need him. They all begin with illusions about themselves and about one another. They all expect to be tortured and mistake one another for the torturer. Garcin, the journalist and man of letters, Inez, the unmarried woman, and Estelle, who is married, make up the closed mixed group.

After the initial introductions, they make quite a point about choosing the right seats. They talk about how they came to be in this particular group, but when they talk, part of their references are to their past lives, and they intermingle the past and the present in a way that clearly shows that they had not yet done with the past. They feel at first that they have come together by accident, but Inez reminds them at once that they have been brought together for a purpose, that nothing in fact has been left to chance, the arrangements in the room, the heating, the colour scheme. Nothing had been left to chance down to the last detail. 'This room was all set for us. They have put us together deliberately.'

ESTELLE: Then it's not mere chance that *you* precisely are sitting opposite *me*? What can the idea behind it be?

INEZ: Ask me another! I only know they are waiting.

ESTELLE: I never could bear the idea of anyone's expecting something from me. All this made me want to do just the opposite.

INEZ: Well, do it. Do it if you can. You don't even know what they expect.

ESTELLE [*stamping her foot*]: It's outrageous! So something's coming to me from you two? [*She eyes each in turn.*] Something nasty, I suppose. There are some faces that tell me everything at once. Yours don't convey anything.

GARCIN [*turning abruptly to Inez*]: Look here! Why are we together? You have given us quite enough hints, you may as well come out with it.

INEZ [*in a surprised tone*]: But I know nothing, absolutely nothing about it. I'm as much in the dark as you are.

GARCIN: We've *got* to know.

INEZ: If only each of us had the guts to tell.

How beautifully Sartre describes the opening session of a group after the introductions are over. Who were they, why were they there, what was the purpose in the therapist's mind that brought them together, what was the guilt and shame, the sin that they were all concealing? Estelle immediately denies that there is anything, and wonders if there hasn't been some ghastly mistake. She hopes that they have made mistakes also with regard to the other members.

INEZ: Is that all you have to tell us?

ESTELLE: What else should I tell? I've nothing to hide. I lost my parents when I was a kid, and I had my young brother to bring up. We were terribly poor, and when an old friend of my people asked me to marry him, I said 'Yes'. He was very well off and quite nice. My brother was a very delicate child and needed all sorts of attention. So really, that was the right thing for me to do, don't you agree? My husband was old enough to be my father, but for six years we had a happy married life. Then two years ago I met the man I was fated to love. We knew it the moment we set eyes on each other. He asked me to run away with him, and I refused. Then I got pneumonia, and it finished me. That's the whole story. No doubt, by certain standards, I did wrong to sacrifice my youth to a man nearly three times my age. Do *you* think that could be called a sin?

The third member of the group, Inez, will have nothing of this. She breaks through the surface.

INEZ: Look here! What's the point of play-acting, trying to throw dust in each other's eyes? We are all tarred with the same brush.
ESTELLE [*indignantly*]: How dare you!

They are still, however, waiting for the official torturer, and Inez guesses that they may perhaps not send one after all. It was an economy of manpower. The same ideas as in the cafeteria where customers serve themselves. The group provides the torture for itself. If this is their aim, thinks Garcin, it could be easily thwarted by their ceasing to communicate with each other, but however silent he can be, the two women cannot keep away from each other. No looking-glasses are provided in the situation, and Estelle uses Inez as her looking-glass. They look into each other, and the reflection they see is more frightening than the one they see in the looking-glass. They have to rely on each other. Inez frightens Estelle by pretending to see a pimple after Estelle has been mean to her. The human mirror can tell lies.

Slowly, but inexorably, the defensive illusions are shed off, and the stark nakedness is revealed. Garcin is no hero, nor is he like a well-beloved brute, as he next thinks of himself; he is a gross coward and very ashamed of it. Inez is a cold-blooded murderer and a lesbian. Estelle drowned her baby. Soon the moment of confession is over, and what then?

INEZ: Well, Mr Garcin, now you have us in the nude all right. Do you understand things any better for that?
GARCIN: I wonder. Yes, perhaps a trifle better. [*Timidly*] And now suppose we start trying to help each other.
INEZ: I don't need any, I don't need help.

Garcin points out how the group integration process is beginning to weave through them, holding them together in a cobweb. 'If you make any movements, if you raise your hand to defend yourself, Estelle and I feel a little tug. Alone, none of us can save himself or herself; we are linked together inextricably.' But Inez cannot see this. How can they help her? And what do they expect her to do in return?

GARCIN: To help *me*, it only needs a little effort, Inez; just a spark of human feeling.
INEZ: Human feeling. That's beyond my range. I am rotten to the core.
GARCIN: And how about me? [*A pause.*] All the same, suppose we try?

INEZ: It's no use. I'm all dried up, I can't give, and I can't receive. How could *I* help you? I am a dead twig, ready for the burning.

How could *I* help you? I am a dead twig, ready for the burning. Garcin points to the dilemma. 'We're chasing after each other, round and round in a vicious circle, like the horses on a roundabout. That's part of the plan, of course. Stop it, Inez. Open your hands and let go of everything.' And Inez asks pathetically: 'Do I look the sort of person who can let go?' Garcin: 'Well, I, anyhow, can feel sorry for you. Look at me, we are naked, naked right through, and I can see into your heart. That's one link between us.' But Inez resents his sympathy and his attention.

The situation becomes more and more intense as they act, interact, react, and transact. Garcin can't stand it any longer and tries to get out. 'I enjoy anything, anything in the way of torture except this agony of mind, this creeping pain that gnaws and crumbles and caresses one, and never hurts quite enough.' He pulls at the locked door with a jerk, and suddenly the door flies open, nearly falling on the floor. A long silence occurs:

INEZ: Well, Garcin? . . . You are free to go.
GARCIN [*meditatively*]: Now I wonder why that door opened.
INEZ: What are you waiting for? Hurry up and go.
GARCIN: I shall not go.
INEZ: And you, Estelle? [*Estelle does not move. Inez bursts out laughing.*] So what? Which shall it be? Which of the three of us will leave? The barrier is down, why are we waiting? . . . But what a situation! It's a scream! We're . . . inseparables!

The group integration process has now proceeded to such an extent that when the doors open, the members find that they can no longer leave. They have to work it out together – the coward, the baby-killer, and the Lesbian. It's no use trying to escape from one anotner. They must try to convince each other. They're inseparable.

Garcin ends the first session. 'Well, well, let's get on with it. . . .'

The uninterrupted, ineluctable group process is seen in all its naked, threatening, and disturbing aspects; the integration proceeds with such rapidity that the recognition of 'closure' is not immediately apparent but then confronts them suddenly as 'a moment of truth'. The effort to open the group fails, and the closed group remains a closed group since its functional closeness has been established, and escape from the internal dilemmas is then seen to be impossible.

4. ARRIVAL AND DEPARTURE OF MEMBERS (OPEN GROUP)

In the open group, the natural history is interrupted by the arrival and departure of members.

The stranger response to new members will be discussed later in Chapter 7 with reference to babies and barnyard fowls, and we shall note Freud's observation that it was very much bound up with self-esteem and the threat to this by anything new or revolutionary. The new member is inevitably a threat and consequently disliked. During the war in Britain, when rail traffic was crowded, there was a cartoon in *Punch* showing a woman and her child struggling to enter a crowded compartment at a railway stop, causing a lot of disturbance to the established members of the compartment. The child remarks to its mother cheerfully: 'Don't worry, Mummy, it will be our turn to hate the next stop.' In the open group, there are many such stops, and, therefore, much hostility is regularly generated. Nevertheless, in serial studies of open and closed groups, it has been shown that assimilation of new members is easier in the open group, although leader-centred and egocentric responses appear to persist longer in this setting. In addition, empathy and related phenomena are less well developed, reminiscence in terms of early life occurs less noticeably except when new admissions or departures occur, the level of group tension and group *esprit de corps* is lower, and specific group phenomena (group dreams, collective fantasies, mirror reactions, etc.) are not so frequent.

The timing for the admission of the new member is an important factor, since a great deal depends on the development of the group at that point. If the group is at a crisis, then a new member may well precipitate a catastrophic disruption, whereas if the group is stagnant, the new member may well prove to be a stimulus for dynamic change. In certain families, difficulties are sometimes resolved by 'getting a new baby', and certain groups similarly rely on 'getting a new member'. It is important before such events are contemplated that the group motivation is fully explored.

The departure of an old member, or his extrusion, also represents a distinctive crisis in the life of the group. Ambivalence once again plays a major part in the group reactions. There is a desire to see the member go as meaning one less person to share the attention, and a stronger desire to keep him with the group because his departure may signify the impending death of the group. In these situations, early separation anxieties, like stranger anxieties with a newcomer, are reactivated, together with guilt associated with the realization of death wishes. Whatever the status of the member, some element of group mourning occurs either in depressive or manic form.

It may be valuable for the group to work through the loss of a member, but once again the timing is important. If it occurs at a time of crisis, it may lead to disruption, but if it comes at a time of stagnation, it may prove a much needed stimulus. Denial mechanisms may also function so that loss may be concealed behind a blank or bland disregard of the incident.

According to Freud, panic reactions are brought about by an increase of common danger or the sudden severance of emotional ties, especially when these take place without warning or preparation. Fear possesses all the members simultaneously, instantaneously, and contagiously, and may lead to chaotic fight or flight reactions. Bion, tying the phenomenon to Kleinian theory, considers rage as important an ingredient as fear, and it is clinically evident that both fear and rage play a part in the phenomenon, sometimes the one, sometimes the other predominating.

The tendency to such panic reactions is closely tied in with what Freud referred to as 'the psychological disadvantages' of being a group as opposed to being an individual. In order to function well, the group needs to develop some of the advantages inherent in the individual. The five principal conditions for doing so, according to McDougall, are continuity of existence, integration, specialization of function, the development of competitive attitudes to other groups, strong emotional relationships between the members, and a shared system of traditions, habits, and customs. Where these conditions are minimal or missing, the 'psychological disadvantages' of being a group come to the forefront, and excessive emotional reactions and inhibitions of intellect occur. The fundamental problem of group life, therefore, is related to the ways and means in which the psychological advantages of individual life can be carried into group life without extinguishing them. It is clear, if one believes this, that in the early stages of a group, the disadvantages will operate until integration occurs and traditions are established.

If we carry the argument a little further, not only is the group at a disadvantage in its early stage of development as compared with the individual, but the artificial therapeutic group is at a disadvantage as compared with the natural group. The therapeutic group is transitional, arbitrarily constituted, loosely organized, tending towards heterogeneity of membership, and summoned together by fate, in the person of the physician, rather than mutual interest. It also has no occupation. In fact, all it has in common at the beginning of its life is its leader and its neurosis. These conditions are optional for the analytic approach, which the leader, i.e. the group analyst, introduces and maintains.

These types of therapeutic groups are therefore liable to manifest 'psychological disadvantages', but, because of the therapist's presence, they never really get out of hand. What occurs are sub-panic reactions at any period when the continuity of the group is threatened, its stability disturbed, or its established structure impaired, without adequate preparation or warning. In such circumstances there may be an upsurge of unstructured hostility blindly directed, of neurotic dread, of a transient loss of conviction about the group process accompanied by cynicism and scepticism, absenteeism, weakening of all group ties and chaotic attempts at restitution. The group for a period seems to be out of control and the therapist experiences it as such. It seems to rush hither and thither without direction, and all ongoing, developing processes are brought more or less to a standstill. The phenomena may be dramatic or sub-clinical and are more characteristic of closed than of open groups. After a period of 'psychological disadvantage', the advantages of the group are reasserted, and the panic reaction is overcome. These advantages include feelings of 'togetherness', 'belongingness', mutual support and protection, alleviation of personal guilt, enhancement of sublimations, and the experience of tolerance and understanding. The 'group defences' create feelings of immunity to the problems that overwhelm the individual, but the defences are less efficient than those of the individual because they have had altogether less time to operate. An upsurge of sex, aggression, jealousy, or frustration may lead to the emergence of the sub-panic reactions.

In the section on phenomenology (page 158 below), the behaviour of barnyard hens with regard to the assimilation of new members is discussed. It would seem that the time interval for assimilation remains very much the same, irrespective of whether the hen is aggressive or passive. Into a mixed group of English people in London, an American was admitted as the new member. The group had been in progress for about two years, and, until this event, had been closed. The group was highly integrated and clearly very resentful when the American appeared, although they had discussed his admission and agreed to it.

In the first phase, the group gave him 'the silent treatment' and took no notice of him except to make cutting remarks and slighting allusions. The American was obviously unused to such an experience, and intruded deliberately and often angrily as frequently as he could. The American, although far from patriotic to begin with, rankled under the general contempt of the group and became blatantly chauvinistic. At one point, when the whole group attacked some aspect of American political life, he became so furious that he began to sing 'The Star-Spangled Banner' to the consternation of the group.

At the sixth session, a new phase began. The American was curiously quiet and was observed to be smiling in a very stereotyped way most of the time. He seemed very unlike himself and was almost manneristic. The group were intrigued but pretended to be indifferent. This persisted for about five or six sessions after which a very curious thing began to happen. The American began to sub-group with one or two of the members and to voice opinions that sounded quite familiar and acceptable to the group. His level of interaction increased, and he was soon very much part of the group, so much so that at one stage one of the members remarked, when he made a tangential reference to his nationality: 'Good heavens, I had quite forgotten you were an American!' At this the group agreed that they never thought of him as such now. He seemed to be just like one of them.

In summary, it is worth recapitulating the phenomena which have a different occurrence in the two types of groups. The process of assimilation is easier in the open group, and the duration of full integration is shorter. On the other hand, leader-centred and egocentric responses tend to persist longer and are reactivated with each new admission. The phenomena of reminiscence and empathy and specific collective dreams and phantasies are more prominent in closed groups in which the level of tension is also higher.

Freud, within the narrow dimensions of his little book,* touches on the problems of leaderless groups, panic reactions, the problem of two psychologies in the group, that of the leader and that of the led, group formations, and group integration. It is, however, group psychology seen in terms of individual psychology. Yet he was more open-handed as regards the possibilities of group psychotherapy than most psychoanalysts are today:

> It appears that when a powerful impetus has been given to group formation, neuroses may diminish and at all events temporarily disappear. Justifiable attempts have been made to turn this antagonism between neuroses and group formation to therapeutic account.

We may well ask ourselves what sort of group therapist Freud would have made. When Kardiner once asked him whether he was a good analyst, Freud is reported to have replied 'No', going on to explain that he was too inquisitive and too patriarchal. These two tendencies would undoubtedly fixate a therapeutic group at an authoritarian level, allowing for very little group development. Had he, therefore, written his *Group Psychology* after a period of group psychotherapy experience, the account would have been substantially the same.

This leads us to the difficulties which beset the psychoanalyst or individual psychotherapist when he is confronted with the group situation.

5. INDIVIDUAL *v.* GROUP DYNAMICS

It is still a matter of controversy as to where one's focus should be when one does group therapy. Should it be on the individual, should it be on the group as a whole, or should it be on the unpopulated region between the members of the group? Some theorists, strongly married to the idea of group dynamics as an end in itself, feel sure that what happens between people is of far

* *Group Psychology and the Analysis of the Ego*, 1921.

greater therapeutic significance than what happens inside them. Others, among whom are especially those who have a large practice of individual psychotherapy, are more likely to regard the group situation as a simple extension of the individual situation, so that they continue to treat the individual in the same way although the therapeutic setting has been changed. The group analyst is, on the whole, less fixated in his focus and constantly shifts his perspective from the intra-individual to the inter-individual sphere depending on circumstances and events. At times, figure is more important than ground, and at times it is the other way round.

The space between individuals is, of course, unoccupied, so that nothing in fact happens there; but if one's psychological antennae are properly attuned to such experiences, the area often becomes 'atmospheric' with feelings. One should stress that this is not a mystical but a phenomenological experience of interacting groups. If one allows one's 'floating attention', as Freud termed it, to record automatically its own observations, one begins eventually to respond to 'pressures' and 'temperatures' as sensitively as any barometric or thermometric gauge with something akin to an internal graph of change on the cerebral 'drum' of the therapist. (If someone could ever devise an infra- or ultra-spectral set of instruments to record such subliminal phenomena and relate them in graphic form to the emergence of content over time, one would have not only a 'natural' description of the group process but also a valuable therapeutic index with information on where the 'pressures' were greatest, when the 'heat' was being turned on, and in which directions the metaphorical 'winds' were blowing!)

Many psychotherapists have combined a practice of individual psychotherapy with group therapy, so that they frequently have to pass from one type of situation to another in the course of a working day. During the individual sessions, they help the patients to re-create their lives from infancy onwards within the treatment setting. When the shift is made to a group session, the time perspective is at once altered. It is almost as if the vertical section of the individual had been cut away leaving the more horizontal aspects of personality. For the individual psychotherapist, the absence of vertical depth represents a loss, but he can be comforted by important gains on the horizontal level.

The couch becomes a panorama and new interpersonal subtleties, over and above transference, enter to enrich the scene.

It is by no means easy to adjust immediately to the shift in perspective, and many therapists are aware of a short phase of readjustment in themselves when they move from one kind of session to the other. For a while, they may find themselves concentrating on the individual and missing all the nuances taking place between the individuals, and in the alternate shift, they may overlook significant transference responses or fail to make some important connexion between the past and present functioning of the individual. It is this peculiar difficulty that occasionally discourages individual psychotherapists from doing group work, and group therapists from taking on individual patients.

Group practice would seem, therefore, to demand a greater degree of flexibility on the part of the therapist, as well as a more constant need for the exercise of his empathy. There are, in fact, more people to empathize with. He has to feel himself not only into the group as a whole but into each individual member, and his sensitivity in this respect will help him to avoid allying himself with one sub-group against another. The sensitivity of the good therapist more or less takes care of such theoretical biases that involve this matter of therapeutic focus. The philosophy in one instance can be summed up as 'what they do between themselves is *their* business; what they do with me is *my* business'. In its other form, this would read, 'If I look after the interpersonal reactions, the individual developments can look after themselves.' A prominent group therapist has reacted to this with the angry question: If the group is doing the therapy and the individual psychopathology is being ignored, why on earth is the therapist being paid? Such subtleties figure more prominently in theory than in practice. One might suspect that the good therapist's attention is an oscillatory one and that the vicissitudes of therapy will largely determine to what extent he is focusing on the group as a whole, on a sub-group, or on some recalcitrant, difficult member. What he does at any particular time is more likely to be dictated by his professional experience of similar situations than to any carefully designed policies of intervention. It would, in fact, be difficult to maintain a dichotomized interest since both individual and group are vividly present all the time, challenging the therapist to ignore their respective needs. To put the matter more simply: when a spectator watches an exciting foursome at tennis, he will be able to follow the flight of the ball from one side to the other, the activities of the individual players, the interaction between the two teams as well as the interaction between the partners depending on his experience with the game and his own ability to play it well. If his capacity for multiple attention is highly developed, he may eventually enter the game as the fifth important member, that is, the umpire.

6. THE PSYCHOLOGY OF THE LEADER *v.* THE PSYCHOLOGY OF THE LED

The problem can be looked at in a different way from the point of view of the individual patient. To what extent does he develop a group as opposed to an individual form of reaction? To what degree does his psychopathology impose an egocentric perspective on him? How much does his individual psychopathology pattern the life of the group? The last question can be extended to include the psychology of the therapist. Once again, there are theorists who look upon the group developments as something quite autonomous once the collection of individuals has become a group. On the other hand, there are theorists who view the history of the group in terms of an emergent evolution in which a large variety of factors, the strongest being that of the therapist, interact to determine the further course of the group. They believe that matters cannot be left wholly to the group and that the therapist must be constantly vigilant in his direction of the group. What he thinks and what he feels will chiefly determine what therapeutic use the group makes of the group. The course of treatment, according to them, does not represent 'a natural history' in its stricter sense. It is a contrived circumstance deeply influenced by the way in which the therapist sets out to 'manage' the group. In the course of treatment, the therapist creates an instrument of therapy with two prongs, one represented by himself, and the other by the group. The therapist becomes more therapeutic for any particular group as time goes on, and the group becomes more therapeutic for itself. The therapist learns to understand and treat the group, and consciously (and less consciously) deploys his own feelings and reactions as therapeutic measures in the service of the group. The therapist does not express these feelings; he is merely sensitively aware of the quality, quantity, and direction. He constantly matches his own reactions against those of the group, just as he matches his background in group experience, his capacity for intuition and empathy and his specialized knowledge of individual behaviour. He cannot overlook these attributes nor can he wilfully decline to make use of them. It is true that he is a member of the group, but a very special one. He participates in the life of the group but in a more complex way. He has to watch his own reactions, his reactions to individual members, and his reactions to the group as a whole. His insight into his own feelings he will keep to himself; his insight into the individual reactions he will make use of to increase his understanding of the group as a whole; and his insight into the workings of the group as a whole he will interpret to the group. As a result of these group interpretations, the group will become more sensitive and sophisticated about its functioning; the individual members will become more insightful about their individual reactions within the group, and finally, the deep unconscious segments of personality will gradually rise up and become more accessible to consciousness. A group therapist has, therefore, no need to make himself into a patient, and the patient has no need to make himself into a group therapist. Both can function fully and successfully in their treatment worlds without encroaching on one another. In this context, the learning to become a good patient is as important as learning to become a good therapist. There are resistances that work against both processes, and these need to be overcome if the cooperative venture is to succeed. As each member of the group develops his own special sensitivities with regard to himself and with regard to the group, the total life of the group becomes, at once, more complex and varied.

If any polarities or dichotomies need to be preserved in group treatment, the differentiation of therapist from patient would make a major claim. In his original appraisal of group psychology, Freud made reference to the two psychologies present in any group – the psychology of the leader and the psychology of the led. From this point of view, it is not sufficient to regard the therapist's contribution as one among several others within the general interactive pattern. What gives any particular group its idiosyncratic flavour is the interaction of the therapist's psychology with the psychology of the member patients. The group, even in its most advanced state, never quite loses sight of the presence of the two psychologies, and although there is a frequent pressure on the therapist by the patients to become a patient like themselves, there is also a concomitant fear that he may do so and allow them to degenerate into a 'leaderless' group, searching for salvation by themselves, yet burdened by all the regressive, destructive forces working with baleful purpose within them. The group cannot treat itself adequately by itself, but it can treat itself more than adequately with the help of the group therapist.

Chapter 7

The Phenomenology of the Group Situation

The data for theorizing on group dynamics are present in all types of groups. Its availability varies from group to group. In some it is cloaked in convention and formalism resistant to any inquiry, whereas in certain mass demonstrations, spontaneous phenomena may be evoked in a profusion that is equally apt to defeat analysis.

In the therapeutic group the uncovering process is not only permissible but pertinent and expected; and in the analytic variety it can be carried out with a minimum of interference and distortion of the material. It should be emphasized that the spontaneous dynamisms observed in the treatment situation exist in all other life groups. Group-analysis does not create them, but it renders them manifest and susceptible to closer investigation. The results of such investigations can, therefore, be applied, with some reservations, to non-clinical groups, and expanded, perhaps, into comprehensive, social theories. It is the group analyst's conviction that he can procure *field* data not otherwise available to the social scientist. He would, therefore, welcome some reciprocal arrangement whereby, in return for the facts supplied him, the sociologist would feed back theory into the therapeutic situation and so enhance its already rich potentialities.

The easy criticism generally levelled at clinical research of this sort is that the experimental field is far too contaminated by the therapeutic aims of conductor and patient to be scientifically serviceable. Although the group therapist does not achieve, or wish to achieve, the simon-pure requirements of the laboratory situation, his 'field' is simple enough in its essentials to allow for endless repetition by many workers. Employing a similarly constructed situation, different analysts have reported the occurrence of similar phenomena, and the emergence of similar predicted phenomena.

No one pretends that this modest arrangement fulfils the rigorous criteria for a scientific experiment. The situation is fairly constant but by no means standardized. The multiple variables are neither described nor controlled, and antecedents and consequents are often related firmly to each other within the limits of chance. But here we are set between the proverbial horns. Too much science will kill therapy; too little science will reduce it to the status of faith-healing. The therapist must steer an uneasy course between the two, trusting to his scientific training and experience to keep him off the rocks. He must place himself in a position to exploit the conditions fully, both for therapy and research, and must deem it unsatisfactory or unethical to practise the one in the absence of the other. Therapy, like motivation, must be included in the experimental field and made an integral part of it. In psychological research, it is now possible to bring in many factors once looked upon with some suspicion as experimental 'contaminants'. The inclusion of these 'contaminants' has given recognition to the complexity of human behaviour. It was only by an exercise of gross over-simplification, based on models derived from physical research, that the human organism could be regarded as an isolated 'stimulus-response' reactor.

Another 'deplorable' tendency the scientists have detected in the researching psychotherapists is a predilection for analogical reasoning. The therapists are roundly accused of amassing their data to test, not operational hypotheses, but analogies, and more often than not, mythologies. It is not sufficient, say the scientists, to claim that a patient behaves in approximately the same way as King Oedipus of Thebes; one must be able to make hypotheses about him which are testable. Otherwise the statement remains, at best, an elaborate and colourful description giving ancient support to thin, modern ideas. We do not here intend to discuss the importance of the myth in the formulation of current dynamic psychological theory. The myth is a timeless concept, epitomizing huge sections of 'deeper' and more 'collective' human feeling. There is no mythology equivalent to the analytic group to help in summarizing experience, and so it is left to us to do the best we can by describing, in faithful detail, the recurrent phenomena that appear in the group therapeutic situation.

The Phenomenology of the Group Situation

1. SOME GROUP SPECIFIC FACTORS

With the development of a group formation, certain phenomena arise that make a specific contribution to therapy in groups. They do not appear in the situation of individual psychotherapy. In addition to these group-specific factors for therapy, there are group-specific phenomena, which result from the workings of the therapeutic process.

Socialization through the group. Socialization is a factor in the human environment that operates throughout life. No one can be an 'island' and, therefore, no one can escape the modifying influences of the society in which he lives. Nevertheless, because of deep psychological disturbances, an individual may feel isolated and inadequate in any group situation and may constantly seek to evade it. A circular response is established; the more inadequately he behaves, the more inadequate he feels; and the more inadequate he feels, the more inadequate he consequently becomes. Society shows itself increasingly intolerant of his neurotic shortcomings and may eventually refuse to accept him altogether. He may then reject society and become a recluse, and the lack of social interaction may lead to egocentric thinking and eccentric standards, which may finally necessitate his admission to a mental hospital.

The 'symptom tolerance' of any given culture may be considerable, but it will still fall far below the tolerance of a therapeutic situation.

In the therapeutic group, acceptance is the keyword. The rejected and isolated are brought in on equal terms. The cardinal lesson of social living is gradually learned – the reciprocal need to understand and be understood. The group listens with patience to the inarticulate, and helps towards a clearer formulation of his problem. It brings him to realize that he is not alone in the absurd, obscene, or incongruous impulse or thought. Much anxiety and guilt are alleviated and long bottled-up feelings find release.

With increasing socialization, the character of intercommunication changes. What was egocentric and leader-centred becomes altruistic and group-centred; references to 'I' and 'me' alter to 'we' and 'us'. From being rigid, absolute, and repetitive, communications become plastic, relative, and modifiable by group experience. Information and explanations are interchanged. The silent members gradually find their tongues and the conversational monopolists are subdued. The value of talking for the sake of communicating is realized. One of Freud's patients referred to it as 'chimney-sweeping'; the accumulated soot in the ivory towers is swept clean.

Therapy lies at both ends of the communication process. We have been talking so far of the transmitting end. At the receiving end, the listeners' threshold for reception is variable and may be affected by any of the hundred and one physical or psychological distractions that habitually block the logical process of thought. The incoming idea may be distorted out of all recognition by the inner circulation of fragmentary phantasies, and lead to misunderstandings and misconceptions. The assumptions or preconceptions, based on the individual's 'framework of reference', may conduce to a personal manipulation of the group material to the bewilderment of others in the group. The amount of distortion is related to the individual's adaptation to reality.

The 'mirror' phenomena. The group situation has been likened to a 'hall of mirrors' where an individual is confronted with various aspects of his social, psychological, or body image. By a careful inner assessment of these aspects, he can achieve in time a personal image of himself not grossly out of keeping with the external and objective evaluation. He can discover his real identity and link it up with past identities.

In the development of a baby, the so-called 'mirror reactions' help in the differentiation of the self from the not-self. The reflections of the self from the outside world lead to greater self-consciousness, so that the infant Narcissus eventually learns to distinguish his own image from that of other images. The mirror reactions are, therefore, essential mechanisms in the resolution of this primary narcissism.

It can be assumed that a member of any therapeutic group has had a disturbed emotional upbringing, and that a good deal of narcissism belonging to his infancy still continues to function in his adult life. The mirror reactions in the group help to counteract this morbid self-reference. By sympathizing and understanding, by identifying with, and imitating, by externalizing what is inside and internalizing what is outside, the individual activates within himself the deep social responses that lead to his definition, in the first place, as a social being.

But if the patient sees himself more and more in and through the group, is there any likelihood of a 'comic' distortion of the self-image as a result of neurotic reflections from the group? Experience has taught us that the image given back is surprisingly true to life. Neurotic distortions tend to cancel out and the composite reflection approximates to the image obtainable in a normal group. The conductor in the therapeutic group can also be relied upon to give back a true image.

The 'condenser' phenomena. The term 'condenser' phenomena is used to describe the sudden discharge of deep and primitive material following the pooling of associated ideas in the group. The interaction of the members loosens up group resistances, and there is an accumulative activation at the deepest levels. It is as if the 'collective unconscious' acted as a condenser covertly storing up emotional charges generated by the group, and discharging them under the stimulus of some shared group event. The discharge, taking the form of group dreams, fears, or phantasies, contains an element of surprise, because of the absence of conscious causal relations. This phenomenon bears some relation to Bion's 'emergence of the basic assumptions' and to Ezriel's 'common group tension'.

The 'chain' phenomena. 'Free' association is an integral part of the psychoanalytic technique for penetrating the unconscious strata of the mind. For obvious reasons, it cannot be used in a group setting. On occasion, however, the group gets near to it in its own characteristic 'free-floating' discussion. This may frequently, in a well-established group, show bursts of chain activity, each member contributing an essential and idiosyncratic link to the chain. The chain phenomenon makes its appearance at certain tense moments in the group, when some 'collective condenser' theme is released – for example, fears of being laughed at, of being neglected, of being victimized. Each member may cap an association with his own. The event can deepen the level of communication in the group and lead to dynamic group developments. It is wiser for the conductor to refrain from joining the chain, since his contribution may bring it to a premature halt.

Resonance. The phenomenon of 'resonance' is another analogical term derived from the physical sciences. The genetic theory of psychoanalysis supposes in every normal individual an orderly development through certain 'psycho-sexual' stages. When something interferes with the developing process, the individual may either revert (regress) to an earlier stage of development, remain fixed at the level at which the interference occurs, or show evidence of precocity. The 'fixated' or 'regressed' person may later enter a therapeutic group and there become associated with others functioning at different levels of the psycho-sexual scale. Each member in the group will then show a distinctive tendency to reverberate to any group event according to the level at which he is 'set'. For example, to use psychoanalytic phraseology, the same circumstances may activate one member to a breast reference, another to reveal his excretory preoccupations, and still another to manifest anxiety over possible injury to his body, and so forth. The deep, unconscious 'frame of reference' is laid down in the first five years of life and predetermines associative responses from then on. The extent of this predetermination can be vividly demonstrated in the group situation.

2. SOME GROUP PHENOMENA

Theorizing. Every psychotherapeutic group starts its life in an atmosphere heavy with theory of a highly fictitious sort. These fictions have already played decisive roles in the life histories of the patients, and the latter cling to them for neurotic reasons. They form a compromise structure related to the degree of genuine knowledge for such 'unknowables' as birth, sex, death, etc., possible or permissible to the patient. They are pragmatically 'true' for the level at which the patient wishes to function.

These theories correspond to the developing child's many theories about sex and reproduction. Both theoretical and factual data is often denied the child, so that its speculations are grounded on phantasies and scraps of knowledge and experience surreptitiously gathered. Educationists frequently discuss the 'dosage' of knowledge suitable for the child at different ages or stages of development. Too little given too late is considered worse than too much given too early. In the latter case the excess is not assimilated. The child's emotional needs at any time govern his requirements, and, understanding these, the best course is to let him work through his infantile theorizing whilst not denying him the right answers to any questions that he brings himself to formulate.

The fictions of the adult neurotic patient in the group represent acceptable causality and are based on a nebulous admixture of conscious and unconscious belief. He may believe, for example, that the war or the housing situation or a mother-in-law may have engendered his symptomatic state, and he may believe this tenaciously because of a temporal association at the onset. He is generally not sufficiently sophisticated before treatment to separate the predisposing from the precipitating cause, and he is especially prone to place his faith more in the single and sudden cause than in multiple factors producing a gradual effect over a period of time. The theory of *trauma* or shock always makes an immediate appeal to patients by virtue of its convincing simplicity.

The therapist has a better understanding of aetiological factors than the patient, but he knows that it is useless to attempt to transfer his knowledge to the patient didactically. Such intellectual insight is soon forgotten because it does not 'belong' to the patient. It 'belongs' to the therapist. The truth comes best in little pieces, slowly but surely, and with the emotions fully engaged in the acquisition. Only then is it properly assimilated. The corrective experience is the result of interaction in the group, whose collective knowledge, reaching into both conscious and unconscious sources, is greater than that of the individual. There is also less resistance to information derived from one's peers, although, on the surface, they may be greedy for 'expert' (that is parental) knowledge. When knowledge is conveyed by an authority, it may be greeted with scepticism, cynicism, or resentment. The conductor on his side must learn to tolerate defective knowledge patiently and sit on his wisdom. His business is not to teach but to assist the group in its learning. Self-knowledge is painfully and slowly acquired. There are no short cuts, although good therapy helps to accelerate the process.

The fiction does not represent merely a stage in the dialectical movement towards fact. It is itself a rich storehouse of unconscious material belonging to a *psychic reality* that is the sum total of the conditions imposed by his inner world on the activity of the individual, which may be meaningful, explanatory, and dynamic in terms of the patient's neurosis. Starting, therefore, with the patient's personal theory, and accepting it as a good working hypothesis, the members grope their way forward into knowledge compatible with reality, or backward into the patient's neurosis. Both are valuable therapeutic experiences, and neither is wholly intellectual or emotional, but a combination of the two. A good deal can be learned from mistakes provided one is not in too much of a hurry to correct them.

Support. Support in the group implies much more than a bolstering up of inadequate feelings or of ideas of inferiority. Abetted by the group, the individual finds courage to express hostile and sexual thoughts that would normally undergo suppression. He is ready to attack because he no longer expects annihilation. He is more prepared to throw down his precious and private ideas into the arena and do battle for them. In the permissive and secure atmosphere of the group, he may let down 'the iron curtain' of repression and expose his vulnerability. He acquires a new flexibility of purpose and the boundaries of his personality are constantly under revision. These deep pressures may lead to softening of the self-lacerating neurotic conscience (the super-ego of psychoanalysis) with a genuine reconditioning of this structure. Such modifications may occur under special circumstances in ordinary living, but in the powerful forum of the group-analytic situation, these influences operate all the time. Patients, under the pressure of insight from the therapeutic process, may resist knowledge because it is painful to know. This was why they buried their knowledge in the first place. The group supports the individual in his fundamental struggle with himself to face the real meaning of his neurotic conflict and identify himself with it. In so doing, they take over the complex role played by the analyst in individual psychotherapy. This represents a peculiar transformation and dilution of the transference phenomenon of psychoanalysis. The group absorbs a good deal of the feeling transferred on to the analyst in the psychoanalytic situation. This is an important function of the group; the time element alone would hardly permit the working through of a transference relationship between the therapist and any one group member.

The tolerance of the group also allows the individual to play the roles to which he is accustomed in his daily life. The capacity for role-playing varies with each individual and the role may not be very obvious. The group will soon diagnose the habitual or favoured role of a person, and by its interpretations bring about favourable changes in role activity. The parts played – that of the favourite, the attention-seeker, the deputy-leader, etc. – attempt to exploit the group situation for some personal advantage and are indicative of the emotional currents at work in the group.

Sub-grouping. The splitting up of the group into smaller fractions forms interludes in the evolution of most therapeutic groups. Every now and then, under the pressure of some tension, there occurs a redistribution of emotional feeling. The sub-group or pair may temporarily cut itself off from the total life of the group. Transient affinities, based on sudden sympathies, empathies, or even on such accidental factors as the sharing of the same public transport before or after the group, may operate for a few sessions. These may lead to further extensions outside the group hour resulting in much privately shared experience and interchange.

The more enduring types of sub-grouping stem from strong identifications, mutuality of symptoms, complementary temperaments (dominant–submissive; introverted–extraverted, etc.) or from feelings displaced from the conductor on to a member. Someone may take a less articulate or adequate member under his wing and speak up for him in the group, defending his interests or protecting him from the attacks of the others. He may also use the silent one as a medium for voicing his own less acceptable views. Such 'projections' may in time be resented by the 'dummy', who may begin to protest, and, in this way, to find his own voice and opinion.

Most sub-grouping resolves itself with the further development of the group, and the conductor, in general, refrains from intervening, unless it establishes itself too strongly and becomes an obstacle to the progress of the group. A mature group, by its understanding and interpretation, can bring to light and resolve these sub-groups, and thereby further the solidarity of the whole group.

Silences. Young groups are often afraid of silences and do their best to avoid them. They learn to depend on certain members who can be relied on to fill the gap. Behaviour during a silence is often strained and anxious. Glances are avoided, and there is an increase of small movements. Members frequently have highly personal and characteristic modes of giving expression to their anxiety.

Silences represent an important communication in the group, and the therapist must endeavour to understand the many different meanings. There has already been a reference to beginners' silence, which, but for the conductor's gentle and tactful handling, would lead to panic reactions. There are silences that follow the release or relief of tension, silences that herald a group 'storm', and silences that follow some deep interpretation of a group event. There are benign silences, brooding silences, perplexed silences, and explosive silences.

Men, on the whole, seem more at ease with silence; women's groups are especially prone to 'defensive' talking – 'tea-party talking' as one group referred to it. Nervous laughter may affect a group during a period of silence, like the irrepressible laughter that grips one during some solemn ceremony. One patient became a prey to incongruously obscene thoughts at such a time and would bend over helplessly to stifle the compulsion to reveal them to the group. Words were used by her to hide her thoughts, and without words her thoughts seemed naked and unprotected.

Silences often mark the end or the beginning of a new phase in the treatment; when everyone takes a breath and waits for the next subject to come up. They look around anxiously for the 'ice-breakers'.

The conductor, understanding the significance of a particular silence, should feel at home in it. His calm acceptance of the situation will help to rob it of much of its anxious tension.

Scapegoats. 'Scapegoatism' is a regular phenomenon in all therapeutic groups, and this raises the interesting question whether or not every group needs, and out of its needs creates, a scapegoat upon whom it can project all its accumulated guilty feelings.

The choice of a scapegoat may depend partly on factors in the group and partly on certain elements present in the chosen individual. The group, in history and in therapy, attacks the scapegoat, because they are afraid to attack the person on whom their feelings are really focused. Analysis of the scapegoat situation reveals this shift of feeling from the conductor, and the transference to him of the extremely mixed feelings originally centring on the father. Groups in which the phenomenon operates strongly contain individuals who have inherent difficulties in expressing their aggression and guilt in the open forum. They project their inner feelings on to some likely recipient, who submits to the projection for inner reasons of his own.

The scapegoat may be selected in the first place on the elemental basis of being different. He may be isolated because of differences in age, sex, religion, class, race, etc. In a well-selected group (see Chapter 3), this is less likely to be the case.

The phenomenon is precipitated when the urgent need for the group to punish meets an urgent need in a particular member to be punished. It is the conductor's task to help the group to recognize its unconscious intentions and so forestall the extrusion of the innocent member.*

The stranger. The 'passing stranger' in anthropological literature was often seized and sacrificed, because he was a representative of the corn-spirit, or was thought to practise the magic arts. In many circumstances, there were elaborate taboos on intercourse with him. The stranger was, therefore, looked upon as a potential threat. So it was with the history of the race. With the history of the individual, there is something not wholly dissimilar.

Until the age of seven or eight months, babies show a friendly or neutral response to strangers. Round about the eighth month, although there are large variations, a reaction sets in. They 'freeze' at the sight of anyone new, and then begin to cry. In the second year, the reaction may be more tempestuous and may take the form of violent screaming. There is then a gradual modification in the response, but even in adult life there will still remain spontaneous manifestations with regard to the stranger ranging from marked hostility to strong acceptance.

A celebrated philosophical controversy of the eighteenth century centred on the problem of the 'stranger response' among primitives. If two primitive strangers – noble savages – were to meet

* F. K. Taylor and J. H. Rey: 'The Scapegoat Motif in Society and its Manifestations in a Therapeutic Group', *International Journal of Psycho-Analysis*, vol. 34, p. 253, 1953

in the forest, the savants asked themselves, would they greet each other with affection, attack each other with hostility, or pass each other by in silence? Today we would be inclined to say that this would depend on what sort of babies they had been, and to what sort of culture they belonged, but at the time of the debate the concept of innateness was not in question. The argument concerned itself with the specific nature of the innate response.

An attempt was made recently to solve the problem in the modern manner – by direct observation of farmyard hens. A strange hen was introduced into a group of hens (New Hampshire Reds). She was a hen with a submissive personality – if hens can be credited with personalities. Within ten minutes she could be spotted clearly as being different from the others. She remained longer in one spot; she moved faster; she alternated statuesque postures with sudden scurries; she remained under cover more and avoided the other hens especially at the feeding trough. She acted as though she was under constant threat of attack; but she ran before she was struck, and she never fought back. Her flighting responses lasted acutely for the first half-hour. For the next few days she was still identifiable by distance and demeanour, but by the tenth day she had blended beyond recognition with the group – a full member, sharing, in close proximity, the feeding trough and the water fountain.

Another new hen was an aggressive hen. In striking contrast with the first, she passed the acute initiating phase in a series of battles, taking on hen after hen, and frequently drawing blood. She showed no signs of avoidance until the seventeenth encounter, which was also her first defeat. Thereafter, her behaviour assumed all the characteristics of the previous hen – scurries and stops, furtive pecking from the floor, and runs to cover. By the tenth day, she, too, was completely blended with the group.

It seemed, therefore, that the 'stranger response' remained the same whether the new hen came in fighting or fleeing, dominant or submissive. The behaviour of both became stereotyped and distinct, and the blending process took about the same time. There was thus a natural period of assimilation which was not affected much by events or personalities. Once assimilation was complete, the new hen entered a second biosocial phase during which her permanent status in the 'pecking order' was established;

that is, she was required to learn (from experience) whom she could peck and who could peck her.

However, hens have small brains and short memories. The 'new hen' in the human group presents a much more complex pattern of response. Basically, as in the farmyard, there seems to exist the same urgent gregarious desire to belong, however distorted this may appear at times from the influence of past experience. In the most asocial and antisocial individuals, one can discern the wish, which is tantamount to saying that, fundamentally, man is a group animal. The stranger in the human group feels the rub of strangeness until he finds acceptance and can blend with his surroundings. The next newcomer reactivates the past uneasiness and challenges the present familiarity with his obtrusive strangeness. It is disturbing to the self-satisfaction of the group, and they must deal with it either by assimilation or extrusion. The persistence of strangeness is intolerable to the group.

Freud, with his customary insight, had something to say about this phenomenon:

> In the undisguised antipathies and aversions which people feel towards strangers . . . we recognize the expression of self-love, or narcissism. This self-love works for the self-assertion of the individual and behaves as though the occurrence of any divergence from his own particular line of development involved a criticism of them and a demand for their alteration. . . . In this connexion men give evidence of a readiness for hatred and aggressiveness, the source of which is unknown, and to which one is tempted to ascribe an elementary character.

In the therapeutic group this 'elementary' response can be followed through its various vicissitudes. It has been found that the rate of assimilation is not as fixed as in the farmyard, and is dependent on many factors. It varies, for instance, with the nature of the group, its homogeneity, the amount of preparation made for the advent of the stranger, the personal qualities of the newcomer, the type of therapeutic environment from which he comes (individual or group psychotherapy, hospital or private practice, psychoanalysis, etc.), the duration of the group, and the readiness of the newcomer to accept the initiation demands.

At a deeper level, the advent of the stranger into the group probably harks back to an earlier situation, when the new baby was first introduced into the family. The jealousy reaction to this has complex determinants, the main factors being the attitude of the parents to the newborn, and their handling of the other children. In the therapeutic group, the conductor is held responsible, as in fact he is, for the newcomer. If he tries to mitigate the 'stranger response' unduly, by helping the new member to talk, or by showing a special interest in him, he may provoke a strongly hostile reaction in the group. The rate of assimilation should be left to the group.

At times, the stranger may defiantly accentuate his difference, so that it appears as a threat to the traditions of the group. The group narcissism is evoked and the implied criticism is taken very much to heart. The members set about changing the stranger or, failing this, changing the group. This may lead to a dynamic shift in the therapeutic situation, so that a protracted stalemate may give place to new moves and new therapeutic openings.

The historian. In the life history of any group, circumstances being propitious, there may emerge a member showing a special interest in and concern with the past history of the group, often to the very minutest detail and often with an avid attention to dates. He is there to remind the group of what has gone before, and to compare and contrast the past with the present. Like certain historians, he manifests, on analysis, a disposition to manipulate the events of the past to demonstrate an undesirable and retrogressive movement away from a 'golden age', when the group situation was altogether much better.

In many respects, the group historian is often as necessary to the group as the scapegoat. He fulfils a real dynamic function. His emergence, as with the scapegoat, depends on a complex of factors, some to do with the group, and others to do with the individual himself. At the time when the historian emerges, the group is generally in a state of great resistance to therapeutic advancement, and has for the time being abandoned, with every sign of inner panic, its forward-looking perspective. Among them is an individual ready and willing to deal with this crisis. He shows an intense neurotic interest in the past (displaced from his own past to the group's past), and a decided capacity for investing it with a nostalgic attractiveness that, in the face of current difficulties, the group may find irresistible. For many sessions, under his aegis, it may 'wallow' in the past.

Such history-making is more characteristic of the 'slow' open type of group, when the arrival of a new member may stimulate the 'historian' (or the group to a less marked extent, since all are potential historians) to reminiscence. It is a defensively regressive phenomenon.*

Rhythm and tensions. Every psychotherapeutic group develops in time a characteristic rhythm of its own. For a time the group may seem to be moving along on dynamic wings, and the members leave the sessions in various states of elation. Not long after, it may give the impression of being at a standstill. Nothing apparently happens, and the members are bored and disgruntled and talk of leaving the group.

There are disrupting and integrating forces in every group. In social groups, the latter are encouraged and the former denied, so that the movement is steadily towards greater integration. Social groups do disrupt, nevertheless, because the suppressed disrupting forces start an underground movement of their own.

The psychotherapeutic group makes it its task to expose and analyse both friendly and hostile elements. Its aim is not integration. It works best at a level of tolerable tension and instability, but the group can tolerate these therapeutic levels of tension only over certain periods. Thereafter, resistances grow, defences operate, and a period of integration sets in. This basic alternating rhythm of static and dynamic, of pause and movement, of rest and change – the Yin and Yang of Sinic Society – has been regarded by Professor Toynbee as the basic process in historical development. All natural institutions to some extent reveal the challenge and response theme which brings about change. In the group, this is self-generating. Each session brings its own dynamic challenge – a new member, an absent member, a sick therapist, a latecomer, as external provocations; the internal stimuli are equally effective.

There is never any need to push or pull the group along. It moves at its own tempo governed by a constellation of forces, progressing and regressing, integrating and disrupting, ceaselessly opposing change and ceaselessly changing, never the same.

> You cannot step twice into the same river; for fresh waters are ever flowing in upon you. . . .

* Cf. page 180 below.

said Heraclitus. And so it is with groups. It is never the same group twice running.

Like all experience, these phenomena – a selection from many that exist – cannot be understood wholly from reading about them. Our social scientist must experience them before he begins to make his theories.

3. INDIVIDUAL PSYCHOPATHOLOGY AND THE GROUP TRANSACTION*

Dynamic differentiation. The group situation can be as effective in exploring the psychopathology of individuals in the group as it is in analysing abnormal behaviour of the group as a whole. Abnormal group dynamics are likely to occur when a normal group is subjected to abnormal stress or when a group is made up of abnormal individuals. In the latter case, the individuals will both behave abnormally, as well as create abnormal patterns of interaction.

The advantages of the group approach to psychopathology are manifest. The investigator is able to study greater numbers at the same time, compare and contrast the cases simultaneously, and watch them 'act out' their psychological impulses in a 'real life' situation and not merely report them.

Whilst the 'mirror reactions' throw more and more light on different aspects of similar symptoms, group interaction may throw more and more doubt on the apparent similarity of the symptoms by referring them to different levels of development. In this respect, the group can function as a deep-going instrument of diagnosis. An illustration of this will put the matter more clearly.

A group was made up of a number of mothers with a single distressing symptom in common – a fear that they might impulsively harm their children, to whom they were otherwise devoted.

This is not an uncommon psychiatric symptom, but each of these women, prior to their group experience, felt that they alone in the world were obsessed with this very unpleasant idea. It seemed to them, and to those who knew them, out of keeping with their kind and somewhat timid personalities. This in part was their solace. Between the impulsive thought and the act there was a

* This section should be read in relation to Chapter 10 where such phenomena are by contrast considered from a new point of view which places the group situation in the centre of theory.

'gap', and the more 'isolated' the thought, the more immersed it was in surrounding mildness and submission, the wider the 'gap' appeared to be.

It soon became clear in the group that the cases were not as homogeneous as they seemed to the diagnostician referring them for treatment. They could be roughly separated into two main types – those who were more depressed, and those who were more obsessional.

The depressed members were less tolerant of the group situation and a few of them left in the early stages. These were unwilling to share the therapist, wait their turn in the group forum, or interact with the other members, except when the problem discussed was very near to their own. They were quite unable to listen sympathetically to any alien experience. Their communications were egocentric in the extreme. On the whole, they were not very popular, and, curiously enough, they appeared to resent this. Their case histories told of an unhappy, neglected, or rejected childhood. They seemed savagely hostile to their mothers or to their memories of them. Many of them had suffered from depressive illnesses, some associated with childbirth. The 'gap' in these cases seemed to be less wide. They were habitually tense, irritable, and resentful, easily provoked to the attack, and punitive with their children. What they thought in cold blood and what they did in hot blood bore a recognized relationship to each other. They came for help, but were disinclined to accept it. One could call them deeply frustrated individuals, who were exquisitely sensitive to any frustration. They were guilt-ridden as a result of their intense inner feelings, and tried hard to compensate for them. They would do things to make their children happy and then envy them the happiness. They often made comparisons between their childhood's unhappiness and their children's happiness.

The obsessional members suffered from an excessive 'house-pride' that made them self-exacting polishers and cleaners for the best part of the day. They maintained submissive, dependent, and apparently good relationships with their mothers, and carried this dependency into marriage and the therapeutic situation, using both husband and therapist as substitute 'props'. In the absence of their 'props', they were liable to acute panic attacks and this gave them a good excuse to remain irrevocably bound up with their 'props' to whom, however, their feelings remained 'mixed' or ambivalent. They differentiated clearly between the cold-blooded thought with which they were at times obsessed, and the hot-blooded act of beating their children when they were naughty and deserved it. They made stable and popular group members, swallowed most of their feelings of resentment, and established polite but lively relationships with each other and with the therapist.

It was clear that in both sections of the group, the impulse towards their children derived from their own childhood impulses but arose from different levels of development. It was not the primary business of the group to connect up the adult level with the level of childhood, but this idea of linking up was eagerly accepted by the group, who saw more sense in it than in linking up with each other.

In the group-analytic situation, the intense dependency needs of the patients made them more leader-centred than was usual even with hospital groups. However, the most dynamic group mechanism was the interaction between the two sections of the group – the depressives and the obsessionals. The former were irritated by the apparently 'good' life situation of the latter, and envied them with the intense feeling that they envied their own children their happiness. The obsessionals, on the other hand, were often alarmed by the narrowness of the 'gap' between the thought and the act in the former. These two basic interactions began to shed a great deal of light on the causal factors in the aggressive impulse and its relation to the 'neutralizing' sexual impulses with which some of the obsessional group were also afflicted. The group as a whole were perplexed by their differences from 'normal' people. They inferred that 'normal' women may occasionally have similar thoughts, but far less frequently, far less consciously, and far less intensely. They concluded that they had 'sticky' minds that retained thoughts that fled evanescently through the minds of others. This was a group-derived theory – part of the therapeutic theorizing that plays a part in the curative movement in all groups. The battle of the 'gap' that went on in this group was the central dynamic group issue. It brought both sides face to face with each other. The 'narrowing' and generalizing of the 'gap' in one case was necessary to counteract the denial of the aggressive feeling and its isolation; the 'widening' of the 'gap' in the other case was necessary to bring the patient back from her deep phantasies to a sense of reality. In the real world, as opposed to the phantasy world, such thoughts are never carried into action.

Significance of syndrome for selection. One could very quickly come to the conclusion that everything is of crucial importance in group therapy, and this comes nearer to the truth the more one becomes aware of the effects of even minute details of structure and function. As in every branch of knowledge, however, some hierarchy of importance does exist. Seating arrangements, the distribution of sexes within the group, the number of patients within the group, and so on, are among the many features that are certainly important, and significant influences belong to the workings of the various diagnostic syndromes that the patients bring in with them to a particular group setting. Neuroses, psychoses, and psychopathies may all exert devastating effects on the life of any group, which is one good reason why close considerations of psychiatric categories are important in the matter of selection. According to some authorities, too wide a range of diagnostic reaction types may build up into a self-disruptive force. Implicit in this concern is the belief, well-founded on experience with social groups, that homogeneity of age, sex, class, race, and religion enhances group formations. Bringing compatible people together certainly makes for a more comfortable group life, but whether it makes for better group therapy is only to some extent true. Many experienced therapists prefer to work with wide ranges of compatibility verging towards incompatibility, since many of the nuclear problems of life stem from an inability to cope with incompatibilities arising out of differences of sex, age, and personality reactions. It is not merely that individual members have to learn that it takes all sorts to make a world or to learn to live with all sorts of people, but more specifically, to learn that he himself has never resolved certain problems of early family life related to differences of sex and age.

In selecting cases for group psychotherapy, most group psychotherapists are probably more influenced by psychopathological appraisals than by psychiatric labels, that is, they are less inclined to worry about patients being neurotic, psychopathic, and psychotic than by the nature and intensity of their basic conflicts. These provide more dimensions to an individual than a simple label which may even work against a proper understanding of his idiomatic maladjustments. There are occasions, however, when the psychiatric nose proves more discerning than the psychotherapeutic one and might lead to the exclusion of a potentially disruptive paranoid individual.

There are some group interactions which appear to have their genesis in the diagnostic syndromes that the individual patients bring with them into the group. We have already discussed the phenomenon of resonance, where individuals at different points of developmental fixation reverberate in a manner specific to the stage to which they belong. These individual vibrations, set in motion by a common stimulus, create a sort of contrapuntal effect. The overtones add a peculiar richness to group life occasioning cross currents of argument, surprise, incredulity, opposition, and interest. It is as if a player, habituated to the narrow range of a single instrument, was suddenly and unexpectedly confronted with a symphonic extension of his little theme. At these moments in the therapeutic group, a sudden widening of the psychopathological horizon may lead to significant group developments. Not only are the instinctual expressions in this complex response different and varied, but the habitual defences associated with them are also manifold. In one group setting, a 'dirty' joke set a series of defence mechanisms into action. One member was quite silent, but disgust showed plainly on his face. Another protested that this was going too far and refused to take any part in the proceedings for a while. Another said that she could listen to these jokes quite comfortably because they aroused no feelings whatsoever in her. Still another respondent attempted to divert the matter into quite a different channel. When challenged about this, he said, 'Whenever someone says something dirty, I like to come out with something that is clean to wipe it off.' A member sitting next to him nodded sympathetically but added that doing this was never sufficient for him; he always wanted to wash out his mouth and hands as well. Such group transactions, therefore, represent a hotch-potch of denial, repression, suppression, sublimation, reaction formation, and protection, the preferred defence once again being characteristic of a particular patient. Out of this variety of defences, a group may develop its own repertoire of defence mechanisms, reflecting such variables as the social class, educational background, previous therapeutic experience and diagnostic category of the individual members. The defences of dominant members may often predominate, and the group may also defend itself collectively against disturbing content or affect. In psychotic or borderline groups, the defence transactions are frequently on a primitive level so that the disturbing stimulus is treated in unrealistic fashion by rapid alternating internalization and externalization, blatant denial or bizarre symbolization. Very occasionally, a collective delusional idea may develop.

In addition to these transactions relating to drives and defences, there are response patterns in which certain psychopathological components seem to play a crucial role. The possible number of such transactions is myriad, but a small sample will serve to illustrate their nature. It is characteristic of such transactions to be complementary, that is, they help to complete each other in a total response. Secondly, since they are latent in all members and manifest in a few, their repeated emergence serves to sensitize group consciousness in this area. Thirdly, transactions within the group are closely reflective of reactions within the individual which are also of a double nature. In individual psychotherapy, the two elements that constitute the whole provoke each other continually so that response cycles are set up in the individual. When a group setting is provided, the response cycle set up in one individual may be completed in another.

Voyeurism and exhibitionism. The therapeutic group is especially susceptible to the development of exhibitionistic-voyeuristic transactions. The arrangement in a circle is designed to show as much of each person to his neighbour as possible. Nothing is provided with which to screen the body or its movements. The same applies on the psychological level. There is a demand for exposure – for the uncovering of one's feelings and one's impulses. It is not at all surprising, therefore, that the latent impulse to show off becomes manifest and is responded to by the latent impulse to look. It is also not unexpected that in group therapy many patients for the first time become aware of such feelings and the ways in which these have affected their behaviour. They become part of that treatment-induced neurosis without which resolution of emotional disturbances cannot occur. The analytic transference neurosis is an example of such a development in individual psychotherapy, and something of the same kind also makes its appearance in group psychotherapy. This is not to say that such a thing as a 'group transference neurosis' occurs, but that certain neurotic developments are brought into the open as a result of the interactive process. In certain instances, a transference neurosis may develop in certain individual members, mainly in relation to the group therapist.

In the mixed group of about a year's duration, three members underwent a spontaneous and temporary sub-grouping. They had found in one another a mutuality of interest that for a period was strong enough to exclude the other members of the group and often reduced them to the role of the silent spectators, interested but not involved. Of the trio, one was a man with a strong clinical voyeuristic tendency who had been referred for treatment because of this symptom; the second was a man whose voyeurism had only become apparent during the course of treatment; the third member was a woman whose presenting symptom had been attacks of uncontrollable and unaccountable weeping, and whose dramatic lachrymations had disturbed and bewildered the group for some time. At the start of the present episode to be described, the woman had had one of her crying attacks, and the manifest voyeur immediately made the accusation that the weeping represented a method of seeking attention. 'It is like showing off,' he said, 'just like the way you sometimes sit with your legs apart.' The woman responded to this observation by recounting a recurrent masturbatory phantasy she had had since childhood in which she imagined herself urinating in front of a large group of people. This linked up the weeping with her urinating and was based on the unconscious belief that the discharge of a large amount of water might create the illusion that a sizeable organ was producing it, that, in fact, she had a male organ. Deep down, she knew that she had nothing much to show from a genital point of view, but during masturbation she saw herself urinating in a sitting position with a well directed stream. She confessed that she sometimes had tried to urinate standing up, but this had been unsuccessful, and she was unable to incorporate it into her phantasy. As usual with many symptoms, a paradox was involved. Whilst calling attention to the man-sized stream she could produce, she was, at the same time, admitting that she was a poor, helpless woman crying out for assistance. At this point, the manifest voyeur recounted a dream of his mother as a phallic woman. In the dream she was naked, dry and dehydrated, somewhat resembling a skeleton, which was in keeping with her real life role of an unwarm person who had nothing to give and whose masculinity contrasted with the passivity of her husband. In his associations to his dream, he disclosed the information that he had never been able to convince himself, even during sexual relations with his wife, that women were 'like dolls' in their physical development. He could seldom bring himself to look at his wife's genitals, but when he did so, he felt that he was unable to distinguish the wood from the trees because she had so much pubic hair: 'With that amount of pubic hair, there is no saying what you mightn't find.'

The woman group member interpreted the dream and his association as a reassurance on his part that she did have a male organ, and she responded positively to the support that he seemed to be giving her. However, her satisfaction was short-lived, because he turned and said to her immediately: 'Of course, it's rather stupid. I know that you haven't got anything to show, but I admit I would like you to show what you have got. I don't think that we need to pretend in this situation.'

The latent voyeur, who was sitting next to the woman, now interrupted to say that he had quite lost interest in having the girl show what she had, and was much more interested in the man showing what he had. He was afraid, however, that it would be much bigger than his. He was against exposure, since if they all 'put their cards on the table', it might well emerge that he had no 'trumps' at all.

One of the silent members now burst in on this triangular discussion. He was a gross stammerer whose difficulties in articulation were accompanied by curious tetanic movements of his protruded tongue between his lips. In the past, this had reminded some of the members of a male organ, and, in general, they disliked watching him in the throes of a stammer because of this suggestion. During the interchange, the stammerer had become increasingly disturbed at what was going on, and his face looked drawn and anxious. Eventually he was able to say that all of this brought back a memory of a long-forgotten phantasy he used to have as an adolescent of girls dancing naked in front of him whilst he masturbated. However, they always had their backs turned to him so that he was unable to see what was going on in front. He was able to reveal this for the first time without stammering and without protruding his tongue convulsively between his lips.

At each stage of this encounter, the wish to see and the fear of looking, the wish to show and the fear of showing something inadequate had reverberated among a susceptible membership taking form in phantasy, dream, and memory. The exhibitionist was provoking voyeuristic responses in the voyeur, and the voyeur was provoking exhibitionistic responses in the exhibitionist. All the responses were interlinked and interchangeable.

Hetero- and homosexuality. Another type of complementary transaction relates to the balance of heterosexuality and homosexuality in the individual. Once again, the setting is a mixed neurotic group in which the inevitable bisexual conflicts of the neurotic individual begin to have repercussions on his peers. Over a period of time, the heterosexual and the homosexual interest appear to take turns in predominating.

It was Freud's belief, as expressed in his *Group Psychology*, that heterosexual impulses within groups lead eventually to disruption, whereas homosexual ones brought about cohesion and integration. The experience of the group therapist would, on the whole, tend to confirm this observation, with the addendum that the two sexual modes are often reciprocally related to each other through an ongoing process of provocation and defence, the one leading to the other in an endless and subtle sequence.

The contributors to this particular illustration included a withdrawn, 'shut-in' young woman, a man, A, with a limited sexual interest in women, and a man, B, who frequently chose to sit next to him. To the surprise of the group, the woman, who had previously often stressed a coolness towards males, began to elaborate a neurotic phantasy about A that appeared to indicate a strong heterosexual attachment. She made great ado at the beginning of each session about whether she should sit next to or away from him. The rest of the group shifted from an early interest in the affair to a later exasperation with her maidenly titillations and panics.

A was both embarrassed and flattered that she should focus this attention upon him, and admitted that it gave his ego 'quite a boost'. Very soon, however, he began to feel threatened with its intensity and persistence. He complained that she was trying to use him to further some heterosexual development in herself. He said that it felt like being swallowed up by a whale, and talked in a somewhat primitive way of being engulfed in the dark inside of this impetuous young woman. Eventually, he even produced a classical 'vagina dentata' – a phantasy of women with teeth in their vagina that could bite off the male organ. He introduced some impressive citations from the literature describing the toxic effects that menstruating women could induce in unsuspecting men. He recalled the fear engendered in him by his menstruating mother and the attacks of diarrhoea that he attributed to her touching his food. A friend of his, who was a physiologist, had reinforced his anxiety by telling him of acid secretions put forth by the woman that could macerate the male organ.

B gave a close and sympathetic attention to these disclosures and declared that menstruation had been one of the most alarming discoveries he had ever made in his entire life. As a small boy, he had accidentally come across a used menstrual pad, and this had been such a shock to him that for a long time he had refused to go near women or even think about them. They had seemed like a terrible and alien species who should have been made by law to carry a red flag signifying danger!

The two threatened males were drawn together in the face of the common enemy and began to show a lively interest in each other. They agreed that they had a great deal in common, and this led to an exploration of overlapping concerns. At this point, A had a dream in which B and himself were on the top of a mountain trying to keep each other warm whilst a dreadful snow blizzard was beating down on them. B's reaction to the dream was immediate. 'Oh, goodness,' he said, 'we were behaving like a couple of old homosexuals, weren't we?' A reddened and looked extremely disturbed by the interpretation. For the rest of the session, he went out of his way to be pleasant to the woman who had showed interest in him. He began talking about having her as a girl friend when the group treatment was concluded and was even tempted to go ahead and ask her out for the evening. However this, he thought, might prove detrimental to treatment, and so after much sober consideration, he decided to postpone his heterosexual intention. For some time after the three members fluctuated between heterosexuality and homosexuality, any forceful expression of the one tendency inevitably serving to drive the individual into the opposite sexual camp. At a later stage, A did bring himself to go out with the woman member, yet the effort was doomed to failure, and both came back to another homosexual sequence in the group.

Sadism and masochism. The sadist-masochistic transactions are among the most 'inevitable' of all these group mechanisms. Once again, an example will best demonstrate their nature. The protagonists in this episode are S and M. S is a highly aggressive woman with a biting tongue which she can use with the effectiveness of a lash. She is rigid, self-righteous, moralistically Victorian, and painstakingly didactic. She is forever trying to teach the group about virtue being its own reward. At times, her sarcasms are extremely cruel. It takes her very little time in the group to discover M's extreme timidity and submissiveness. His vulnerability is a constant provocation, and on many occasions she turns the group situation into a Roman holiday, subjecting him to a merciless attack. He makes little attempt to escape from this predicament, and his remarks frequently seem designed to antagonize his assailant further, although made with an anxious watchfulness in her direction. The constant repetition of the pattern brings the mutual tendency into the open, and she begins to accuse him of deliberately provoking her in order to bring down her anger on his head.

He becomes equally well aware of this and attributes it to the fact that this reminded him vividly of his mother: 'My mother treated me in very much the same way. Whenever I said or did anything that was in the least contrary to her expectations, she would lash into me and make me feel like a real worm that deserved to be grounded to the earth. I so began to expect her attack that when she failed to make it I would feel as if there was something missing and work hard at provoking her.' S was stung by the comparison: 'I'm just tired of being everybody's mother. Wherever I go people will try and make me into their mothers, and I'm going to tell you here and now that I am just not going to be your mother.' But become his mother she gradually and inevitably did. They set up their own little sub-group and limited the interchanges to themselves. Every now and then he would cringe beneath the sarcastic barrage. A silence would then develop between them until he set off another attack.

After a while, M brings out some hidden phantasies about being beaten and tortured, and S reacts to this in characteristic fashion:

'So that's what you're after. You are trying to make me into a torturer so you can get a kick out of it. Well, I am not going to play your game. The last thing in the world I want to become is a torturer. I am not going to torture you, however much you want it.' But torture him she does, week after week and month after month. It is with some satisfaction that M remarks: 'We do make a peculiar couple. You want to attack, and I want to be attacked. It's as simple as that. We might as well get married.'

The night after this remark, as if to demonstrate that such situations are far from simple, M has a dream in which he has tied S to a wall and is beating her while she is complaining: 'You can't do this to me; I'll tell Dr A about you' (Dr A being the group therapist).

The reversible positions of torturer and tortured become clear to the group, and once again the sequence of phantasy, dream, and memory set the manifest and the latent in juxtaposition so that the complementary features of the transaction are at once discernible. At the end of this particular session, S remarks: 'Isn't it funny! Here we are talking about who is being tortured when really we are all being tortured by you (Dr A).' Here she generalizes from her own sado-masochistic tendency to the group as a whole. The patients are all there to suffer, justly and inevitably, at the hands of the sadistic therapist. The whole treatment process is no more than a sadistic-masochistic transaction. The model of the treatment situation in the first illustration based on the exhibitionistic-voyeuristic transaction is of patients exposing themselves to the voyeuristic therapist; in this model, they are being sadistically punished for their wrongdoing. The analysis of the group model built up on the latent inclinations of the individual members is a potent therapeutic procedure. Treatment cannot help but uncover and cause suffering, and patients can make use of these inherent aspects to further their own pathological needs. Inevitably they will see the therapist as pruriently curious and his interpretations as onslaughts which they need to endure. A typical group dream envisages the therapist as a lion tamer battling ferociously with his lions but always in command because he has the 'whip hand'.

Male–female competitiveness. The fourth transaction is inevitable in a mixed group. It concerns itself with the basic human situation of sex difference and the interplay of feeling between the 'haves' and the 'have nots'. The neurotically exaggerated pride of the male provokes the neurotically exaggerated envy of the female, and the ensuing conflict tends to focus on the rivalry between the sexes, at first on a manifest level, but eventually deepening to an unconscious level.

A, a male patient, has taken up flying with a great deal of enthusiasm and is anxiously working towards his 'wings'. He is constantly informing the group of his progress, and it has become quite a group joke. Since this is a group well on in its therapeutic development, its members are able to point out A's need to demonstrate his masculinity, and in this they are not far off the mark. He is indeed very much concerned with his ability to be potent with women. He suffers inordinately from what has been described in the psychological literature as 'the small penis complex', and he spends a great deal of time with a measuring tape, but the measurements never satisfy him. He is sometimes 'amazed' by what he surreptitiously glimpses in men's lavatories, and it depresses him. He is anxious to take the women members of the group flying with him, and with a certain amount of sly amusement, they respond to his invitation on two levels. Could they trust him whilst he was still unlicensed? Would he be able to keep them 'up in the air' all by himself for so long? Was he certain he knew his way around the controls, and that he could handle them efficiently? Couldn't they have a go themselves? To all this, he would answer furiously and literally. They had to come as his passengers, since this was the rule of the club. It took a lot of experience to handle an aeroplane, and women were quite hopeless about machines. His solo experience was sufficient guarantee that he could fly passengers. He had been up as long as two hours by himself.

B is contemptuous about it all. He sees it as just a substitute for the real thing. He doubts very much whether flying can make you feel any more potent. You might jump over a six feet wall to get to a girl, but the problem of what you did when you got there still remained. He feels strongly that you have to do things directly and not beat about the bush. He tells the group stories of extraordinary sexual feats, adding that women in some countries have been given medals for multiple motherhood, and he saw no reason why men should not have visible insignia of some sort that would indicate their capacities. The women in the group react in various ways, some accepting his stories and others preferring to regard it as pure phantasy. To this B replies that he would like to prove it to them and let deeds speak louder than words. 'But it's one of the rules of our therapeutic group that we can't have such demonstrations,' comes the reply. One of them remarks that B reminds her of Don Juan, and that her understanding of this adventurer, if the psychology books meant anything, indicated that he was only an impotent homosexual striving to prove himself a man. It was because he was so inept that he was driven to promiscuity and boastfulness. At this interpretation, B turns on her angrily and says: 'Whether we have three women each night or not or whether we can fly fifty miles or not, at least we've got something that you haven't got. Put that in your pipe and smoke it.'

The battle between the sexes. The battle between the sexes is on, and each side becomes increasingly provocative. To one particular woman who is reacting with great intensity to every male attack, B remarks with cutting emphasis: 'It must be terrible to sit over there and feel that you have nothing to show at all.' She looks outraged. 'What do you mean, nothing? You are just biologically illiterate. We've all got something. It just happens to take different forms. The mass of apparatus is the same; it is simply a question of visibility.' B, who is leading the male attack, shakes his head. 'You can't call what you've got *something*. You yourself know it's nothing and that's why you are so prudish.' The women squeal in unison, and one of them goes on to say: 'That's where you're so wrong; it's not nothing. It's something that makes the world and keeps it going. Where would you be if it weren't for that something? Put that in *your* silly little pipe.' Another adds: 'What's more, we've got things that you haven't got. We've got breasts which you haven't got. We can produce babies and feed them which you cannot do. We are self sufficient, but you have to depend for everything on us.' A hears this with disgust: 'That's just what you'd expect of women. They're so irrational. Whenever you've proved to the hilt that they've got nothing, they try to show you that they have twice as much, which is silly.'

At this point, the women tire of the biological argument and turn to everyday life. Their leader is venomous about the two men. 'Both of you are really failures as men. There isn't enough masculinity between you to carry you anywhere in the world. That's why you both live in a world of phantasy. The difference between you and us is not a question of what you've got and what we haven't got, but of our being successful and of your being unsuccessful.' There is a large measure of truth in this remark, the women in this group being better educated, better paid, and having higher community standing than the men. The men are reduced under this new attack to a state of silent, sulky depression. She goes on: 'It's not we who are jealous of you; it's you who are jealous of us. We have probably read more books together in the last month than the two of you have read since you left school.' B mutters about 'blue stockings' and then goes on to make a crude comment that she could keep her books between her legs for all it was worth to her. All in all, it is an even battle with both sides very much on the defensive. Eventually, like most group battles, the struggle begins to move in the direction of the therapist. Could he arbitrate in this impossible situation? Could he decide about what was 'something' and what was 'nothing'?

Here again they are confronted with one of those 'givens' of a group situation, the dichotomous model of therapist and group, the basic classificatory difference. The women grumble at the unfairness of the situation, and one of them says: 'Well, he is bound to be on the side of the men, because after all he is a man, he is bound to be against us in this matter.' Talking among themselves, they decide that the only thing they could do in the face of this brute fact is to leave the group and find a woman therapist who worked with groups. The therapist is just as bad as any of the other males in the group. He parades his own maleness with the same blatancy and egotism. The male members, perhaps relieved at finding the attack shifted away from them, cannot identify the therapist with their cause. He is the god who sits by himself and has everything and gives nothing. He is the really potent individual who sees the group as a collection of weak, impotent people. They can now make common cause with the women against this obscene, omnipotent figure, the only one in the group really equipped to deal with all aspects of life in a thrustful, successful fashion; the only well member of the group. The focus has shifted from the psychopathology of the individual to the psychopathology of the sub-group, and finally to the psychopathology of the group as a whole contrasting itself with the therapist, and at this point group analysis and group interpretation become possible. This is one transaction among others. The women do not leave the group, and go a long way towards resolving some of their basic problems concerning envy and pride, while the men concomitantly consider matters of impotence and femininity. Side by side with the envy of the opposite sex come the beginnings of a mutual admiration for maleness and femaleness and the complementary roles of the sexes.

Manic-depressive transactions. These are among the most interesting to be observed in any group. They tend to be set into motion when depressive people become members of a group or when members sustain or imagine that they sustain some catastrophic loss. There is, in addition, a contagiousness in such affective responses as elation and depression, and groups are inclined to be deeply affected by any predominant emotion that impinges on them.

The ingredients of this transaction are made up of anxiety, transient despair, apathetic detachment, defensive excitement, and grief. There is a subtle interplay of elation and depression as they enter into the general matrix of the group's emotional reactions. One sees it especially at times when members leave the group, fall sick, or die.

In the following clinical illustration from a women's group, a woman, C, had just lost her father through death. For some time before his death, she brought bulletins about his condition, and it seemed that she was preparing herself and preparing the group for what appeared to be an inevitable outcome. She was also asking the help of the group in coping with her mounting anxiety and guilt with regard to a period during her adolescence when she and her father attacked each other with unremitting hostility. She had then consciously prayed for his death, and now, twenty years later, the fulfilment had caught up with the wish. She wanted to be rid of all traces of death-wish before his actual death, and she looked to the group to absolve her. The group responded positively to this demand and reassured her that each and every one of them had frequently quarrelled with their fathers many times during their lives, and they felt that her particular case was within the statistically normal range of response. Some of the women had had dreams indicating death-wishes towards parents, and all agreed that adolescents were given to much exaggerated expression and that something said in the heat of anger need not necessarily be regarded as a true index of real feeling. It was not a cold-blooded wish. The woman pointed out that she had made many acts of reparation since those early days. She had frequently given her father money, bought him his weekly tobacco, and lent him a beautiful bed to lie in and die in. She couldn't have done more for him in the past few years without neglecting her own family. The group assured her most earnestly that she had done everything possible to exorcize the evil thought and told her that the good relationship she now enjoyed with her father was proof enough to them that the old demon had been successfully laid to rest. They gave her to understand that when her father died, they would still be there to support her, and she would not lose them however bad her feelings were then or at any other time. There was no doubt that she derived a great deal of comfort from the group's positive attitude towards her forthcoming bereavement. At times, it resembled the solemn and supportive interchanges between women preparing a shroud. There was a profound commonality of purpose.

In the session following her father's death, she arrives in a deeply depressed state completely dressed in black. She gives a sorrowful account of the entire proceedings from death to interment and weeps bitterly as she recalls the sound of dirt descending on the coffin. The group is embarrassed and a little perplexed, as if they did not expect her to show this intensity of sorrow after the work they have put in on her, and there is some trace of impatience in the questions they ask her. They seem curiously aloof to her grief. The promised support in her hour of trial does not seem to be forthcoming. Without any further mention of the death, the women begin exchanging little jokes. The hilarity grows until it almost sounds like an Irish wake. The mourning figure of the sad, silent, and bewildered woman sitting isolated in the group makes the reaction appear even more bizarre and incongruous. At one time, one of the women begins to intone: 'John Brown's body lies a'mouldering in the grave', and no one is disturbed by the fact that it is in such poor taste.

The therapist himself is somewhat perplexed by the group's behaviour and out of sympathy with it. He feels the need for some intrusion into the situation and considers offering some simple expression of condolence to the woman. As if anticipating him, she turns towards the group and says: 'I must thank you for trying to make me feel happier.' The group is startled, and one of them asks rather brusquely: 'Happier about what?' the woman says: 'I mean about my father.' They fall silent, and then the previous speaker says, more gently: 'I am sorry. I am afraid I forgot all about that.' The others in the group echo this in a similar guilty fashion.

Following this session, the woman sets about her mourning in a typically orderly and organized manner, and she takes to bringing bulletins recording the diminution in her grief reaction. First she discards her black dress and then the black armlet; next she allows herself to watch TV and go to a movie; then she feels able to start sexual relationships with her husband; and finally, she is able to report that she no longer has vivid dreams of her father as still alive. There is no doubt that she behaves as if she is very pleased with herself. Her father is now dead and buried, and she is happier than she has ever been before. 'I used to feel so awful about him,' she says, 'but now I can see things realistically.' She becomes increasingly cheerful and, at one point, is described as the 'life and soul of the party'. It is at this stage that the group begin to react to the situation and, once again, the discrepancy of affect between the woman and the rest of the group is striking. She is now oozing gaiety, constantly making the silliest little jokes, and is in fits of laughter over nothing in particular, whilst the rest of the group sit solemnly discussing death and damnation, the possibilities of suicide, the absurdity of life, and their sorrow over the death of loved ones. As she comes out of her depression, they enter into theirs, and at the height of her elation they are like spectres at the feast.

That this is a transactional cycle makes itself clear when she succumbs again to the unspoken condemnation and relapses into a state of depression with suicidal ideas. A more genuine mourning process begins, but once again it is cut short by the counter-reaction of the group. With each transaction there seems to be a working through of the problem and an enhancement of insight. The growth of self awareness is closely associated with the growth of group awareness, and group awareness develops with the activity involved in differentiating the group from the group leader. The group may respond to the leader in numerous ways. They may see him as the powerful healer in relation to themselves as sick, as the normal one with themselves as abnormal, as the parent with themselves as children, as the strong one with themselves as weak and helpless, etc. In the transaction just described, they began to see him as someone immune from emotional provocation, maintaining stability and serenity at a time when volcanic eruptions of feeling were taking place.

In a later session, at the tail end of the manic-depressive transactions, the group takes the therapist to task for not feeling sorry when a member is burdened with such terrible news. They upbraid him for lacking common human feeling. How can he sit there and gloat about his own happy circumstances when they are all so low-spirited. The least thing he could do would be to show some 'professional' signs of sadness. They feel that his happiness, in fact, derives from their sadness and that he has become a psychiatrist in order to derive vicarious satisfactions of this nature. Later when the group reaction lifts, and the state of general euphoria ensues, they mockingly refer to him as 'the undertaker' whose business is death and who has found it professionally necessary to eradicate joy from his life. The analysis of the affective swings of the group in relation to the therapist then becomes the key procedure in the ongoing group movement.

Progressive and regressive forces. One final transaction noticeable in the daily life of the group involves the reciprocal relationship between progressive and regressive forces. Progress, in any particular member of a group, invariably acts as a challenge, a stimulus, or a provocation to all the others, initiating flights into health, flights into sickness, rivalrous claims, scepticism and cynicism, and mechanisms of imitation and identification. There may also be a peculiarly negativistic response to progress by the group as a whole which may sometimes result in gross symptomatic behaviour and 'crazy' histrionics. Each individual seems to take upon himself the historical load of sickness brought in by all the members and his struggles are watched by the group as an epitome of what besets the total group. With the individual, progress may imply the termination of treatment, the severance of established group ties, the loss of group support, and an end to the valuable group life that they have only recently found. The group are quick to differentiate between real progress and flights into health, just as they become experts with regard to authentic disturbances as opposed to flights into illness. The group may react with anxiety to both regression and progression, since the former may signify that they are not doing well and may eventually become collectively mad, and the latter that they may lose each other and lose their therapist as a result of termination of the group. Regression and progression may, therefore, bring into play a series of progressive and regressive defences as counter-balancing measures.

P and S are two women in a group who maintain a close companionship even outside the group and make frequent comparisons about their progress both in the group and outside. The group tolerate the association very well and refer to them as 'the heavenly twins'. At one stage, P loses her job and feels very hopeless and helpless about it. She stays in bed most of the morning and can neither fend for herself nor look around constructively for new employment. At about the same time, S's behaviour in the group is peculiarly triumphant. She has got herself engaged to be married and takes up a great deal of group time planning her wedding and making detailed preparations for the babies that are to follow in regular succession. She is apparently surprised to see P in tears during her recital and makes continuous reference to her new-found health and her readiness to leave the group. Her immaturity, however, does not stand up to the real life situations. Under very distressing circumstances, her engagement is broken off, and a shameful retreat into dependent family life takes place. Her phobias once again become prominent, and she finds it hard to face the group, more particularly her friend, P, whose whole behaviour has simultaneously picked up, and who now lavishes mature counsel on poor S. Her solicitude is unbounded, and she fusses like an overprotective mother. She manages to get herself another job and tries hard to get one for S as well. The alternation of the mother-child roles is circular enough to force itself on the attention of the group, and no one is left in doubt that the two transactors derive a great deal of vicarious gratification from each other's regressions. Eventually one of them is able to remark with insight: 'I'm getting tired of being at the other end of the seesaw to P. I don't want to spend my life just going up and down with her. It's awful to think that I can only be good when she is bad. I want to do much better than that. I want to be good on my own, just because I want to be good.'

The regressive-progressive conflict soon irradiates from the couple to the group, so that the group begins to react regressively to its own progressions and vice versa. The group is on the seesaw with itself. Much of this behaviour becomes clearer in relation to the therapist. He is generally viewed as the embodiment of progression, biased in the direction of maturity, and purposefully and masterfully furthering the healthy features of life. As a mode of rebelliousness, the group will sometimes react to this progressive ideal and indulge itself in gross immaturities. They sometimes behave like small children at a party when the harassed adult is trying to restore law and order. At other times, the therapist is viewed as a hindrance to their mature aspirations. He is driving them back to reconsider their childishness, remove controls from their associations, become more spontaneous and flexible, and in general, loosen up. At these times, the group is defensively adult in its attitudes, and the proceedings settle down to a level of polite tea-party talk. When, on the other hand, he tries to make the group look at itself from the standpoint of its mean chronological age, then they react like two-year-olds. The group is now at the other end of the seesaw to the therapist.

Group dynamics and group therapy. There are, of course, many more transactions than have been reviewed here. The kaleidoscopic pattern of group dynamics is made up in large part by an interplay of such transactions between members, and between the therapist and the group; and only under careful analysis do the various basic components emerge. One should really speak of a transactional complex that dominates group activity at any particular time and is made up of various subsidiary transactions such as those described earlier. It must be also understood that such group dynamics take place within the general therapeutic setting of the group and are very much part of the therapeutic interchange. By abstracting them from their general context, the picture looks more like group dynamics than group therapy, but there is no group therapy without group dynamics, and group dynamics is essential to the understanding of a group therapy.

All this is in keeping with the orientation of group-analytic therapy which is directed towards making the group therapeutic in itself and capable of handling much of the business of therapy largely by themselves. This does not imply self-effacement. The therapist is there to be used when the group needs to use him, and they learn to use him when they cannot reach a satisfactory conclusion by themselves. In the group-analytic session, the intervention by the therapist is chiefly dictated by the needs of the group rather than by the demands of the individual or a particular situation. The therapist is concerned that the group process of therapy should move forward under its own momentum and refrains from interfering with the autonomous developments by keeping too much to the individual requirements or the individual situations.

Like every other ingredient of the group, transactional phenomena may work both for and against therapy. They belong to the latent life of the group and become manifest largely as a result of group work carried out by the group members in conjunction with the therapist. As we have seen in the selection procedure, it is not helpful to balance neurotic against psychotic patients, and this holds true in the psychopathological sphere where one does not select exhibitionists and place them with voyeurs in order to provoke a transaction. This sort of crude manipulation has no place in analytic group therapy. Transient sub-groups are a normal part of the therapeutic life of any group, and one must be wholly prepared for the different symptomatic and functional groupings that take place from time to time. The selection of complementary psychopathological types would create a contrived and artificial atmosphere that would interfere seriously with the spontaneous development of the group. On the other hand, the normal, spontaneous experiences within the group will encourage the emergence of certain repressed characteristics in patients, and it is these latent manifestations that conduce to the complementary reaction. It is not possible or necessary to foresee all such developments, and even if one could foresee their development, it is not necessary to set about avoiding them. Such reactions may from time to time act as islets of resistance within the group, but for the understanding therapist, the moments of resistance are also the moments of challenge which his therapeutic skills are there to encounter and master. The resolution of a complementary reaction often leads to a further consolidation of therapeutic gains within the group.

The group is not always aware of the subtle interplay of action and reaction. Take the illustration of the manic-depressive transaction, for example. The group had been preparing itself for some time to be helpful to the member when the time of bereavement arrived. They had planned to support her, reassure her, and, to some extent, share the burden of her mourning process. But the best laid conscious plans often go unconsciously astray. It seemed at first as if they had forgotten about the woman's predicament or that they had detached themselves from its significance. Certainly, no conventional condolences were offered, and no empathetic depression occurred. There was, instead, a wholly inappropriate response taking into consideration the socio-economic and cultural background of the members. What they did was done without conscious effort or intention and, consequently, they were surprised when the woman thanked them towards the end of the session. They did not realize that their behaviour had been different, and for this reason it is not comparable to the effort sometimes made in everyday circles to counter a period of depression in an individual with an attempt at forced cheerfulness. This was at a different level of functioning altogether. On one level, the group as a whole was refusing to accept death as an authentic experience, and the occasion of death, therefore, served as an existential crisis. On another level, the group was refusing to share the woman's sense of loss, as if to defend themselves against any reactivation of similar experiences in their own lives. Had they been able to react differently, each member might have, in turn, resuscitated some incomplete process of mourning from their past lives. Such incomplete acts of mourning belong to all our lives and serve as depressive foci to which we return from time to time under the pressure of some appropriate kind of stress. At still another level, the group seemed to be punishing the woman for threatening their narcissistic equilibrium and adding to the reservoir of anxiety and depression with which the group had to cope. 'It is bad enough to deal with what we have already inside us; why do you have to bring in still more from outside?' could have been another interpretation of their behaviour. Finally, we have to take into consideration the whole problem of unconscious guilt, the unwelcome member of every group session. Old death-wishes, stemming from earlier conflicts within the family, are prone to make their reappearance when the death of a parent once again intrudes on the neurotic interactions of a group. The unconscious wish: 'I want the father to die because he has frustrated my expectations' is at once matched with a counter-wish: 'The father is not dead; there is no reason for guilt and there is no reason for mourning.'

As might be expected, the resolution of this particular transaction did not take place without the therapist's phantasied death and the denial of that particularly frightening wish. In fact, one might say that whatever belonged to the complex psychopathology of depression was there in the group and that the primitive manic defence constituted the group's only resource at that particular time for dealing with it. At least part of the group's reactions had to do with their interference with the process of mourning. At all times and in all climes, the pattern of mourning has been rigidly ordained within certain temporal limits. It almost seemed as if each culture was sufficiently aware of the psychic status of its members to prescribe an appropriate dosage of grief and restitution. In one of the great Sophoclean tragedies, an interference with the process of mourning becomes the central issue of the play. One must bury the dead in the prescribed manner or else grievous consequences will result.

Chapter 8

Group-Analytic Psychotherapy with Children and Adolescents

1. GENERAL PRINCIPLES

Group therapy with children, like group therapy with adults, can be organized to include a wide range of therapeutic situations, which allows the therapist to prescribe more appropriately to the child's needs. Some types of disturbed children, for example, do better in mixed diagnostic groups, some with groups in which there are mixed sexes, and some in settings where the age range has been stretched a little to include both younger and older children. Again, some children are more responsive when confronted with a group occupation, whereas others will create their own interests and activities or restrict themselves for long periods to purely verbal interchanges. Some of these differences are related to the age and sex of the child, but temperament, personality, and diagnosis also play a considerable part. Having male and female therapists and co-therapists also available serves to expand the spectrum of treatment still further. Although such provisions aim at obtaining the right type of group for the right patient, it is well to remember that selection criteria are, at best, only approximately effective in this respect, and that it may be of more therapeutic worth to allow the individual to adjust himself to the requirements of the group than to find a group that is ideally adjusted to his idiosyncrasies. By concentrating too rigorously on compatible membership, there is a double danger of defeating one of the crucial therapeutic functions of the group which is to resolve disturbing differences or the disturbances associated with differences, and, secondly, of creating a compulsive organization that disregards ends in its pursuit of means. It must be borne in mind that group therapy is still in the fallible stage of learning from its own mistakes and that even if we work towards providing a particular patient with what he needs at a particular time, it is still worth trying him out in a group when age, sex, and diagnostic considerations do not appear altogether promising.

We can now proceed to discuss some general issues with regard to the psychological treatment of young people. It is a clinical commonplace that many children during their development suffer excruciatingly from the stereotype of the child erected and tenaciously preserved by the adults in their environment. A particularly popular one views the child as an immature being whose major problems have to do with being insufficiently adult. This perspective of the young is generally one of amiable condescension that makes allowances for a relatively simple organism, unrealistically and naïvely oriented towards the problems of existence and, like the young of most species, dedicated to a life of energetic playfulness devoid of serious implications. As far as this kind of grown-up is concerned, the 'un-grown-up' individual is an uncommunicative, often unintelligible creature whose actions tend to speak louder than his words, in fact so much so at times that he is preferably better seen than heard. This drive to activity is impressive enough to have led some group therapists, overlooking the presence of other richer proclivities, to emphazise its possibilities as a medium for therapy. In this context, activity may be considered in either a supportive or analytic framework.* In the former, it is regarded as a form of catharsis, whereas in the latter it is viewed as a non-verbal communication that can be interpreted verbally to the child. Inactivity would represent a state of resistance. This is in direct contrast to the situation with adults where action is decried as resistance and the therapeutic aim is to immobilize the adult and compel him to express himself in words rather than deeds. *Verba non facta.* What is, therefore, good therapy, it would seem, in the child becomes bad therapy in the adult, and vice versa. There are no grounds for believing that such a viewpoint is true and that motility means something basically different in the case of adults as compared with children. The group-analytic approach has been to make no such distinction but to focus on verbal expression in both child and adult as the preferred mode of communication, believing that the main technical problem in child therapy consisted not in interpreting activity but in converting it into speech. More so than in the adult, it is

* S. R. Slavson: 'A contribution to a systematic theory of group psychotherapy', *International Journal of Group Psychotherapy*, vol. 4, 1954, pp. 3–29.

characteristic of the child to make use of verbal and non-verbal forms in most of his communications. Sometimes he does both together, and the message is concordant, whereas at other times his activity belies what he says.

To carry out any sort of therapy with children involves a capacity to talk to them, and talking to children requires effort and practice. It is more difficult to talk therapeutically to children than to adults, because it requires more radical change in one's normal talking habits. Since most adult communications to children take the form of information, advice, and prohibition, they are largely one-way channels allowing for minimum feed-back. To establish a two-way communicative process with the child usually necessitates a complete change of attitude and behaviour in the average adult. He must become interested in what the child has to say to him, and since factual information is not the child's strong point, he has to relinquish some of his propensity for 'data-gathering'. He can become interested in the child's communication because it represents an unusual viewpoint of the world seen through a pair of innocent and highly subjective eyes (as in the case of the 'Emperor's New Clothes'), or he can become interested because the child's answers reactivate part of his own childhood experiences and open up, once again, a lost world of childhood. This has circular value. To get back into touch with one's own childhood may be a gratifying experience in itself, but it also is an essential element in the process of establishing contact with the child and developing the necessaıy empathy. This mysterious attribute requires a transient surrender of one's own intrusive adult personality together with an associated regression. It allows one to experience what it feels like to be a child of a particular age and sex looking out at the world without the accumulative experience of thirty, forty, or fifty years. (Fifty is probably the limit since after that the psychological distance tends to become too great for successful therapeutic rapport.) To talk to a child without talking down to him is not an easy matter for many adults. He must be able as a simple requisite to reorganize his phraseology, vocabulary, and grammatical structure in keeping with the child's age without lapsing into an embarrassing 'baby talk'. Given an adult who talks his language, the child is able not only to talk but to talk back. Successful talking with children above all implies reciprocal communication.

An example of good talking with children in groups can be found in any of the early books of Piaget. He began talking to children, in his inquisitive and interested manner, about forty years ago and has continued to talk to them in a way that is never didactic. Nor is the child ever made to feel his ignorance and inadequacy in the presence of an omniscient, omnipotent being who is able so easily to deprecate and disparage his little communications. In this approach, there is a complete suspension of scepticism and unbelief, and under these conditions, the child will open the door to his magical world of childhood and admit the right sort of adult in. There is no 'open Sesame' in the form of some rule of thumb. It is simply a question of the child convincing himself that the adult in question liked, understood, and appreciated children, and was prepared to listen to them. There is nothing specific about the language. In general terms, it is the language of childhood; it is simple, brief, direct, and concrete. It has a starkness which defies artful dissimulation and circumlocution. It attempts to say what it means.

Another feature of childhood to which the adult must accustom himself is playfulness, because playfulness has an important part in any therapeutic relationship with children. The playfulness may take the form of actual play, an enactment of phantasy, or a playful approach to the world of the adult. The child may use it to entertain himself when alone or with others, comfort himself when miserable, abreact himself when tense, and express himself when language is insufficient. In a memorable article, Freud linked the daydreams of the adult, the poetry of the poet, and the play of the child to one another, and in any significant treatment situation there is something of all three present. Whether the child is daydreaming, playing, or rhapsodizing, the heart of the matter is in the stream of unconscious phantasy that plays a vital part in his daily psychological life. For the adult to be playful implies that he has ready access to the same sources of phantasy that nourish the play of the child and, because of this, might be better able to participate with him in the same collective phantasy.

The group behaviour of children varies in the course of their development. In situations of group upbringing, such as in the Kibbutzim of Israel, experience has shown that quite small children, hardly out of their infancy, can already show evidence of group orientation. Toddler groups are, on the whole, loosely structured and ephemeral, but with the onset of latency and active social life, the groups begin to organize themselves in more structured formations. Piaget has called attention to the extraordinary behaviour of latency children who, in order to throw snowballs at one another, will often begin by wasting a quarter of an hour in electing a president, fixing the rules of voting, dividing themselves into two teams, deciding upon distances, and finally framing the sanctions to be applied in case of infringement of the rules. In adolescence, the groups again become smaller, and in later adolescence bisexual groups may emerge.

Age and natural group formation to some extent dictate the therapeutic techniques used with children, and it is essential that the therapist make himself familiar with the developmental phases of childhood and the sequential changes that occur in the intellectual, emotional, social, moral, and linguistic spheres. This presupposes a good understanding of child psychology and development as background knowledge to group therapy with children.

A further important aspect of therapeutic work with children that every therapist must bear in mind constantly is that he is dealing with other people's children, and that other people's children are by definition children who have been brought up in quite the wrong way and have incorporated the more objectionable attitudes and sentiments of their parents! When children are exposed to the *mores* of the therapist, there is inevitably a conflict of loyalties.

The fact that these are other people's children also means that the barriers and taboos are weaker than when we deal with our own children and are, therefore, likely to stimulate more conflictual feeling around aggressive and erotic impulses. In general, there is more counter-transference response in child therapy than in adult therapy, and in group therapy as compared with individual therapy. In doing group therapy with children, therefore, the therapist should expect to experience appreciable amounts of positive and negative feeling that may at times occasion guilt and shame or inadvertently discharge itself on to the children. When recognized and suppressed, the same feelings may find their way out in the excessive tiredness, boredom, irritability, permissiveness, strictness, forgetfulness of names, slips of the tongue, and cancellations of sessions.

Psychotherapy with Children and Adolescents

Based on fifteen years experience of group therapy with children, the author has elaborated three separate techniques in the group-analytic approach to the kindergarten child, the latency child, and the adolescent.* These have been labelled, for convenience, the 'small table', the 'small room', and the 'small circle' methods of analytic group psychotherapy with children.

2. THE 'SMALL TABLE' TECHNIQUE WITH KINDERGARTEN CHILDREN

This method is suitable for children ranging in age from four to six. A small round table was evolved after much experimentation, four feet in diameter and eighteen inches off the ground, the surface of which is divided into five sectors, each separated from the other by a low, removable wall. Between the walls lies the place or 'territory' of the individual group member. The walls radiate to the centre of the table where there is a trough containing water, and each territory has a small area of access to it. The water trough is there as common property whereas the territories 'belong' to the individual members. Each territory is equipped with a set of play things – human figures, animal figures, housing, transport, etc. (the ordinary paraphernalia of play therapy) – and each set has its own special colour, distinguishing it from other sets. The transactional processes in this nursery group are carried out on both the concrete and verbal level. On the concrete level, the children may scale the miniature walls with ladders or tunnel beneath them. They may lend their toy equipment, and in this way help others to elaborate their play themes, and in turn, they may borrow from them. The need to have more space for the realization of their ideas may force the children into a reciprocal 'social contract' with a neighbour. The group members squat or kneel round the table, and the therapist occupies a similar position as a member of the circle, on the same eye level with the group. The therapist has his own territory and play equipment.

In the early stages, territories tend to be respected, and each child cultivates his own area. The play is at first individually centred with little reference to the activities of other children. Soon, however, they start to watch what someone else is doing

* See *Age and Syndrome in Group Psychotherapy*, Journal of Long Island Consultation Center, 1, 2, May 1960.

and may even begin to imitate him. This type of parallel play proceeds for a while until the children get to know and accept one another. 'Communications' at this stage are at the level of the 'collective monologue' described by Piaget. The children talk about what they do and about what it means. The 'running commentary' accompanies their activity and is not apparently directed at any one in particular. Its purpose is not obviously to communicate. Motor activity supplements language to a large extent. Silences are frequent and natural. At this stage, the children are therapist-centred and tend to seek and maintain his attention. They will come around to 'borrow' equipment that they need in addition to their own, and the therapist will try and make the interchange a model for group interchanges. He will 'lend' judicially, because he has to relate himself evenly to the group members. The duration of the first stage varies with different groups. In some the territories remain relatively sacrosanct; barriers are respected and equipment jealously hoarded. From a visual point of view, there is a colour segregation, and each child is strongly aware of his 'colour' and the coloured objects that belong to him 'by right'.

In the next stage, group developments begin. The boundaries between the territories are crossed, and personal play themes begin to encroach on neighbouring ones. At first there may be resistances leading to withdrawal or active rejection on the part of the child whose territory has been invaded, but subsequently a link-up of two play themes often occurs to the manifest pleasure of the participants. As time goes on, more and more linkages are spontaneously evolved, and for a period a single play theme may dominate the proceedings. Visually, a diffusion of colour over the table takes place as equipment begins to circulate to meet the common or mutual purposes. As treatment proceeds and boundaries are removed, the territories are no longer individualized, so that a picture of group integration can be observed in a very concrete and visual way. The various stages of group development can be photographed in colour providing a convenient clinical record for the therapist.

With the coming into being of these spontaneous 'play associations' there is a change in quality of communications. At the height of the play interactions from time to time a 'collective phantasy' is embroidered, a development of the 'collective monologue', each child adding his share under the exciting stimulus of the 'libidinal' material in his hands. These phantasies centre around home situations – the new baby, the aggressive elder brother, the absent father, the possession of the mother, the 'naughtiness' of mess-making and noise-making, and so on. Pleasurable and destructive impulses are mostly directed against the 'good' and 'bad' material, but may easily overflow on to the participants. Most of the quarrels are over the ownership of some material and can be distinguished from hostilities stemming from phantasy.

The therapist, as in the adult situation, is there to serve the children. He participates in the play themes but only passively, adding nothing of his own. Occasionally the children may appeal to him for support or help, but this is mostly in the very early stages. He interprets only in terms of the 'collective phantasy' so that the interpretation is directed towards the activity of the group as a whole.

It is important to work within the limits of fatigue, and thirty to forty minutes is ample time for group meetings taking place twice a week. It will be seen that this type of therapy is very much an adaptation of play therapy and makes significant use of the symbolic content of the play.

An example of collective phantasy. Nursery Group. Average IQ: 115. Type: mixed, fatherless children. Session 5. The children have been in session for about 15 minutes.

ANN [*digging a little horse into the sand in her plot*]: My lovely horse is going under the ground. He likes it there because it's warm. There are nice things there he can eat if he likes to.

MICHAEL [*has been zooming about with a plane but keeping to the boundaries; eventually he crosses over into Ann's plot*]: I'm coming to kill your horse. I'll drop a bomb on him. Look out! [*Ann begins to whimper. Michael continues in a more aggressive tone of voice.*] My Dad can kill everybody. He was a pilot and he killed lots of people. When I'm old, I'm going to be a pilot and kill everybody.

ANN [*defiantly*]: You can't kill my horse, because he's mine. My Daddy gave him to me. My Daddy will kill your Daddy because he's stronger. [*Both fathers were, in fact, dead.*]

JOHN [*to Michael*]: You can come and kill my horse, because he's a stupid horse and has a broken leg. [*John's father had deserted the family when he was a baby. Michael kills off John's horse, but returns to Ann who has her hands over her horse protecting it.*]

MICHAEL [*in a changed tone of voice to Ann*]: If you put him under that box, I can't kill him. [*Ann does so, and the belligerent plane is returned to base.*]

In these group interactions, the therapist does well to keep to the background. There is no need to interpret the Freudian horse. However, the group interpretation of the 'collective phantasy' can be highly effective even in the nursery group. An example of this occurred in a group of four very inhibited and over-controlled children, two boys and two girls, who came to their first group session so immaculate that the therapist was almost inclined to swathe them in overalls rather than risk a spot.

For the first few sessions, there were no group formations whatsoever, no interchange of equipment, no collective themes, and altogether a paucity of verbal comment. It was a very noiseless group, the children being of the kind who are seen and not heard. There was some polite recognition of one another by the sixth session, and in the seventh session Peter found out about the ladders and tunnels and very quietly and somewhat awkwardly attempted to connect up with Janie's territory. Janie was clearly outraged by the intrusion and kept saying 'No, No, No' in a somewhat frantic but stifled voice. Peter's persistence was surprising in the face of her opposition, but he seemed curiously determined to bridge the wall and to stay 'put'. The two children grappled with the bridge, and eventually Peter pushed the dividing wall over. At this point, Janie was so angry that she found nothing to say and just stood still and wet her pants. The three other children were startled by this outcome, and Peter whispered that Janie had made 'pee pee'. The two other children took up the whisper, and soon there was a scandalized whispering chorus of 'Janie made pee pee, Janie made pee pee'. Janie was clearly as dumbfounded as the others since she was not a child given to 'accidents' and had been triumphantly toilet-trained by the time she was thirteen months. Now she stood in a little puddle quite at a loss to know what to do, her expression indicating a mixture of confusion, guilt, and shame. Eventually all she could say was: 'I don't care' somewhat defiantly. The therapist asked her if she would feel more comfortable to change her pants. She went out to the waiting-room and did so but returned quickly to resume her place, leaving, however, the wall down so that she was now in a liaison with Peter.

At the next session there was a radical difference in the group atmosphere. There was a new camaraderie in the air and much of it focused on Janie. There was also more verbal interchange, and, under the stimulus of this, Janie began a phantasied theme, having secured the quiet attention of the other members. It concerned a little girl, a princess, who lived all by herself in the wood and had no playmates (true of all the children in this group). One day she was walking by a pond and accidentally fell in, and soon she was drowning. At this, Peter became very excited and cried out: 'Don't let her drown, Janie. I am coming'; and soon an improvised wooden boat was launched to rescue the princess. Caroline, another member of the group, observed with awe that she was very wet and that she would die because she would get a bad cold and fever. The princess was still floating in the water, and Peter was trying to scoop her up unsuccessfully. Eventually he said with exasperation: 'Everyone can get wet if they want to. She is not drowning, she is floating.' The group seized upon the situation, and soon the pool was full of personnel from different territories, much to Janie's pleasure. The still voice of conscience emerged from Caroline who paused enough to say: 'Won't the mummies be angry?' She was answered by George with a firm finality: 'No, 'cause they're away.' The excitement continued as the boundaries were knocked down, and the equipment put into general circulation, until no sense of orderliness remained, and the group table indicated group integration or disintegration depending how you looked at it; it was certainly a battlefield. It was difficult to understand what the children were saying at this point, since they were all talking together, and no one was listening to anyone else, although the rapport was excellent. The timid Caroline eventually turned to the therapist and with some urgency asked him: 'What are they all saying, Dr A? What are they all saying?' The therapist turned to her and said, quite quietly, 'You know what I think they are saying, Caroline. You really know what?' The group paused at this and looked on. The therapist continued: 'I think what they are saying is it's all right to make a mess and make noise. You don't have to feel bad about it, and the doctor doesn't mind.' Peter's response to this was: 'Hooray for the doctor!'

The breakthrough that coincided with Janie's wetting herself was maintained, although not at the same level of disinhibition. The 'working through' of this critical incident took several sessions and consolidated into a real therapeutic advancement.

3. THE 'SMALL ROOM' TECHNIQUE WITH LATENCY CHILDREN

In an early technique with latency children, modified from Slavson, the activity needs of the children of this age group were taken very much into consideration. A contract was made with the members in the very first session whereby an activity period of their own choosing followed a talking period. The children were generally seen in separate age groups – the five to nines and the ten to twelves. They were run in conjunction with certain occupations such as drawing, painting, or modelling but the sessions were otherwise quite unstructured. The therapist was occupied along with the group, and his productions open to the same free criticism. Mixed groups at the earlier age seemed to do quite well, and active and passive types to blend congenially together. The session ran comfortably for an hour and was rounded off with a short spell of activity in which all could participate. Five or six members made a good therapeutic 'gang'.

The inhibited section of the group were at first passive spectators of the interaction among the active, boastful, and garrulous members, providing them with an audience. Among the latter, there occurred a special sort of child, generally a boy, with a colourful and engaging personality, histrionic to the extreme, and constantly 'putting on an act'. He personified the hero but could be easily identified as a passive, somewhat fearful child who was compensating wildly for his chronic feelings of timidity and inferiority. The heroic disguise was only too easily shed under stress, but under average conditions his bright social intelligence shone through the group and made him both a focus and a target for group feeling. The brighter the limelight, the more was he stimulated, and the more stimulating did he become. He exploited the group in a noisy, blatant, and theatrical fashion, and, in the early stages, undoubtedly helped to integrate the group more rapidly than would otherwise have been the case. His inner disturbance gave him a psychological sensitivity that was valuable for activating the more stolid members. The mercurialism on the face of it looked so much of a group asset that a therapist might be excused for making use of it to get his group going. The disadvantages of this 'stimulator' had to be weighed against his credits. After a while his monopoly of the group time tended to hold up the therapeutic work and direct it away from the 'natural' course of the group.

Eventually the group tended to find him out and to give him back a bit of his own medicine, but by this stage he had often dropped out or been transferred to a newer group where the cycle of events was often repeated with little alteration. The metamorphosis of hero into scapegoat began when the group diagnosed the child's underlying weakness and his refusal to face this constructively.

During the early experimentation with latency groups, the 'discussion phase' was by no means inactive. At this age, it is almost unnatural for children to say what they have to say rooted to a chair. Generally, communications were 'acted out' on the move which meant that the sessions were full of drama and the 'stage' more often crowded with two or three players at a time trying to engage the rest of the audience. The chairs round the table were often abandoned early during the proceedings unless the occupation, if there was an occupation, was of sufficient interest to tie them down. Generally the children fitted themselves into any available nook or cranny, and in the free situation of the group it was almost symptomatic for the unoccupied child to sit down on a chair. In fact, sitting a child down on a chair was a most effective way of reducing him to silence. There were no rules except against vandalism, danger, and injury.

Towards the end of the discussion phase, the group took off some time to choose their activity. It was quite surprising how often the group would spend as much as fifteen of their thirty minutes in group discussion to determine what to do. There was generally relief when the discussion phase drew to a close. The clamour for activity would have begun, and spontaneous activity would be on the increase. During this terminal phase the group would often combine against the therapist as if he were the restraining factor on their more spontaneous behaviour.

These latency groups have a charm and a character of their own. 'Gossip' is their strong point. They enjoy discussing personalities and group relations. They are shy about their symptoms, especially such regressive ones as bedwetting, and they dread losing face. In the later stages, the preoccupation of the prepubertal members with such topics as sex differences, sex roles, the mysterious problems of birth and death, and the fears of calamitous happenings at home is very much in evidence. In the group they defend themselves against such anxieties with much hilarity and noise, and they characteristically lead up to tabooed subjects in a welter of witticisms and elated behaviour. Much of their mixed feelings for their parents rapidly settles on the therapist. The following is an account of two groups run on the contract basis. In this approach, the therapist would be very much a 'participant observer' in the group but would try and keep his interpretative interventions during the discussion phase for moments when the group drama included all the members in a particular 'act' that arose spontaneously out of the group situation. During the activity phase, the activity *in toto* would be interpreted either in terms of the group's needs or as a manifestation of their relationship to the therapist.

The following two accounts are examples of this approach and are a compromise between the activity groups of Slavson and the verbally oriented groups that developed later.

Verbatim report of a latency group (boys). Ages: 10–12. Numbers: 5. Mixed symptom group. Session 9.

This first report illustrates the continuous interaction, the 'acting out', the rivalry between two potential leaders (David and Raymond), and the behaviour of the 'group stimulator' (Raymond) under stress. The group have already 'diagnosed' him. David comes into the room looking depressed and draws comments from the group, mostly positive and sympathetic.

'Gosh, he's got the hump – whatever's the matter, Dave? – I bet he's putting it on.' (At a previous session David had informed us that he could make himself sick whenever he wanted to, thus escaping unpleasant situations.) David ignored this last comment and came and stood by the doctor's chair tracing on the table with his finger. He seemed curiously ill at ease.

DAVID: Doctor, do you mind if I ask you something? [*I shake my head.*] Well, I've been thinking about something and I can't make it out at all. [*He continues to finger the table whilst we all sit patiently.*] You see, my sister's name before she was married is not the same as my name. Why should she have had a different name from me, can you tell me that?

RAYMOND: Well, we don't want to hear about that now. We'll have no time to play in the end. Tell the doctor some other time. [*The interest in this remark lies in the fact that Raymond's father is also under suspicion of not being genuine, but Raymond has never been able to face this at all.*]

JOHN: I bags we hear. It's like a detective story. It's like the films.

DONALD: Give old Dave a chance. It's good to get things off your chest.

RAYMOND: Why should you worry about a name? I've got a funny name, but I don't worry the doctor about it. They used to call me 'greasy' at school because it's a Greek name.

DAVID: It's not like that. I was thinking that my father is not really my father but my stepfather. [*There is a small silence as this sinks in.*]

DOCTOR: Well?

DAVID: Do you know if it's true?

RAYMOND: Why ask the doctor? Why don't you ask your old man?

TEDDY [*speaking for the first time*]: He can't.

RAYMOND: Why can't he? He just hasn't got the guts. He's just a filthy coward.

DONALD: I'm sure I couldn't ask my Dad things like that. He'd wallop me.

JOHN: I'd prefer to ask him rather than my Mum. [*John's mother is an aggressive, masculine type of woman.*]

RAYMOND: Well, it's no use asking my Dad anything because he can't speak English properly.

DAVID: I was going to ask him. I'll ask him tonight.

DOCTOR: How long have you been brooding about this, David?

DAVID: Since before Christmas.

DOCTOR: You mean from the time your mother said you were not so good at home.

RAYMOND [*flippantly*]: You bad little boy. Aren't you good at home then? Don't you look after the baby when you're asked to? I'm awfully good – I do all the housework and shopping at the weekends.

DONALD: Gosh, you wouldn't catch me doing that.

JOHN: My Mum wouldn't let me.

DOCTOR: How is it you kept this secret to yourself for so long?

DAVID: I don't know. I didn't think we had to talk about that sort of thing. I don't know.

RAYMOND [*chanting*]: Don't know was made to know; don't know was hung. . . .

DAVID: Oh shut up, you fool. If you had this sort of thing, you'd worry about it.

RAYMOND: I never worry about that sort of thing. I'd worry if my asthma came back. Ask the doc. I used to worry about all sorts of things but I don't any more. I've finished with all that. I can take anything that's coming now.

JOHN: How do you know it won't come back?

RAYMOND: Because I know. I used to be afraid of scrapping titchy kids. Now I'll bash anyone at school.

DOCTOR: So you think you're better, Raymond?

RAYMOND: I certainly am, and you know I am, Doc.

DAVID: If you're so much better, why the heck do you come?

RAYMOND: That's for doctor to say, so shut your gob.

TEDDY: Go on, hit him.

DAVID [*rolling up his sleeves*]: Well, if he wants to fight. . . .

RAYMOND [*hurriedly*]: I wasn't talking to you in any case, so it's none of your business. I was talking to the doctor. [*Turning to the doctor*] I was going to ask you whether you wanted a bird's egg. [*He offers round little egg sweets; finally to David magnanimously.*] You can have one if you like. [*David appears somewhat overcome by this approach as he accepts one.*] You've got to take me to the pictures one night, though.

DAVID: O.K., we'll go tonight if you've got any cash. [*They take out their cash and examine it.*]

RAYMOND: Twopence short. Doc, if you like me, you'll lend me twopence.

JOHN: Doctors don't give money. They only give medicine and advice. You shouldn't ask doctors. Why don't you ask your Dad?

DONALD: The boot's on the other foot now. I bet he's scared.

RAYMOND [*with disgust*]: Scared! You fools. It's simply that I know that I won't get it from my Dad. I'm not scared of anything.

DAVID: You're scared of me.

RAYMOND [*ignoring this*]: I'm not scared of the doctor. [*Dances up pugnaciously to the doctor and starts to hit him.*]

DOCTOR: Why don't you pick on someone your own size to fight? You don't have to bully me. [*The group all laugh at this and Raymond returns to his perch on the window.*]

RAYMOND [*to David*]: If you ask your Dad about being your Dad, I'll ask mine for the twopence. Still, Doc, you're a bit of a stinker. Anyone would think I'd asked you for a million pounds.

DONALD: I don't think it matters how much you ask for. I couldn't ask my Dad for anything. My Mum's always given me my pocket money.

RAYMOND [*savagely*]: That's why you're such a cissy baby.

TEDDY: Why don't you fight? You only talk.

RAYMOND [*to doctor*]: Doctor, I don't like this bloke and I'm not coming to any more meetings if he's coming.

DAVID: Hooray! Close the door behind you, will you?

RAYMOND: Who says I've gone? Don't count your chickens. [*Teddy suddenly drops a book he's holding on to the floor.*] You see, Doc, a year ago that would have made me jump out of my skin. Now I don't bat an eyelid. That's nerve for you.

JOHN: What's wonderful about that? None of us did. [*Raymond is picking up something to throw at John.*]

DOCTOR: What were you going to say, Raymond?

RAYMOND: I was just going to ask him what he meant by tripping me up in the gym in the last meeting.

JOHN: What did I mean? What did I mean? To knock you down, of course.

RAYMOND [*belligerently*]: You're very lucky the doctor's here.

DAVID [*aggressively*]: So are you.

RAYMOND [*flippantly*]: Well, we're all lucky the doc's here. He's a smashing doctor sometimes, and sometimes he's not. When he makes us talk, he isn't; when he lets us play, he is.

DONALD: No one *makes* you talk.

RAYMOND: You're just jealous because you stammer.

DAVID: I'd sooner listen to Doc any day than to you. At least he always talks sense.

RAYMOND [*to Doctor*]: Why the devil do they always pick on me?

JOHN: We don't pick on you. You stick your neck out. You like to be the centre of things.

RAYMOND: That's a damn lie.

JOHN [*calmly*]: It's only a lie because you don't like it.

RAYMOND: I don't know why I come to any of these rotten meetings.

DOCTOR: *Why* do you come, Raymond?

RAYMOND: Because I want to. Don't you want me to come?

DOCTOR: You're always welcome if you think it helps you.

RAYMOND: Well, it's better than playing with the gang down our street. They're too interested in girls for my liking. How I hate girls! Silly, soppy things! [*There is a chorus of approval over this and Raymond brightens at this. He walks up and down the room miming a girl's supposed type of walk with swaying hips, etc., to the great delight of everyone.*]

DAVID: By gosh, you look just like a girl. Old cissy!

RAYMOND: Say that again and I'll bash you.

DAVID [*delightedly*]: Old cissy! [*There is a brief but pregnant silence.*]

RAYMOND: If is wasn't for this arm of mine you'd have got something. [*To doctor*] Doc, why don't you do something about my arm? You call yourself a doctor and you don't do a thing.

DOCTOR: That's the first time I've heard about your arm. What's the matter with it?

DAVID: Let's see it. We'll put it right.

RAYMOND: You keep off. I want a real doctor.

JOHN: The doctor's a real doctor.

RAYMOND: No, he's only a talking doctor. He only reads stupid books. Like that one in his cupboard *Basic Problems of Behaviour* – you didn't know we had found it, did you? [*Puts on a mincing voice*]: 'The observation of the children should be carried out with discretion and unobtrusiveness.' [*The group laugh uproariously.*]

DOCTOR: What do you think of that, Teddy. Unfair, isn't it?

TEDDY: Give him a damn good strapping.

DOCTOR: What for?

TEDDY: For being cocky.

DONALD [*suddenly*]: I bet that's what your Dad does. It's what my old man would do if I fooled around with him. He makes me stammer badly when he's angry. I talk much better when he's at work. Sometimes when he comes into my room at night to put his overalls in the cupboard, I think I'm having a nightmare, and I get up shaking.

DAVID: Talking about nightmares, Doctor, can you tell me why I keep having the same dream over and over again?

RAYMOND: I've had lots of dreams – just ask the doctor. He made me paint them. Rum things weren't they, Doc?

DOCTOR: Well, tell us about this dream, Dave, and we'll see if we can discover what it means.

DAVID: I'm always walking down the street towards the shops in order to get something for Mum. I want to give her something nice. And I'm always fifteen years old and it's my sixteenth birthday in a few days, and then I get knocked down and killed.

DONALD: Really killed? You can't be killed in a dream. You always think it's going to happen and it doesn't. I always imagine I'm falling down a cliff but I never hit the bottom. But the nearer I get the more scared I get.

JOHN: Perhaps you think your Dad's at the bottom.

DONALD: Funnily enough I never dream of my Dad. I never dream of my Mum either although I'd like to.

DAVID: But I'm sure I must be dead; my legs or my arms are usually chopped off.

DOCTOR: And you never get to sixteen?

RAYMOND: You see, Doc, at sixteen we're allowed to go to 'A' pictures on our own. We're supposed to be grown-up then. I'm dying to get to sixteen.

DOCTOR: So is David apparently.

JOHN: I shall leave school when I'm sixteen, thank goodness.

DAVID: It gives me a funny feeling in the pit of my stomach when I think of this dream. I want to die of heart failure when I'm old.

JOHN: Anyhow it's only a dream, so why worry. It doesn't mean it's going to happen, does it, Doctor?

DAVID: But it stops me from going to sleep. I'm too scared to go to sleep sometimes, in case I have the dream.

DOCTOR: The dream may simply mean that you have some worries about growing up, Davie, and you probably feel that you're not going to make much of a showing. Dreams are not the same as life, and so the same things don't have the same meaning.

RAYMOND: My Mum says it always means the opposite. So cheer up, Dave; you're not going to die. It probably just means you're going to have your hair cut. By the way, Doc, what are you going to let me take away this time?

DOCTOR: I never let you take anything. You just take them. Why do you do it?

RAYMOND: I like pretending, that's all. I always bring it back anyhow, don't I? Could I have your coloured pencil, this time? [*He takes it and the meeting breaks up.*] Doc, I shan't come again if that fat guy comes. Can't we just have you, David, and me?

DOCTOR: I thought you didn't like David.

RAYMOND: I don't, but you do, so I suppose he's got to come.

DOCTOR: Well, I'll see you next time. I must go and have my tea.

RAYMOND: Eating again. Fatter and fatter. You get more like my father every time I see you. You'll soon be just like him. Then he can come and take the group and you can come home and live with us.

DOCTOR: That mightn't please your mother.

RAYMOND: But it pleases me and that's what matters.

Report on a latency group (*boys and girls*). Ages: 9–12. Mixed symptom group. In-patients from a psychiatric ward, Maudsley Hospital. Session 7.

The late latency group does very well when the sexes are mixed. This group met three times a week and occupied themselves with drawing. The report gives evidence of the teasing kind of chatter that so characterizes these groups. The preoccupation with sex differences, sex roles, birth and death, and growing up is manifest. The tendency to defensive pairing up of the two girls, so typical of this age, is associated with an indignant 'masculine protest'. Eric is a 'stimulator' and functioned in exactly the same way in another group to which he was transferred. Vivienne's strong interest in killing is not accidental. It repeated itself from session to session. Her mother had been murdered a few years earlier under very curious circumstances. Father had remarried and

Vivienne's behaviour corresponded to that of a female Hamlet.

The overtones from the adult world are always there. At times the conversation does suggest the world of 'miniature adults'.

Doctor, Eric, Vivienne, Barbara, Rosemary, John. [*They settle down to painting.*]

ERIC: The doctor is a saint. St Anthony, don't you know.

ROSEMARY: I want to sit on your lap.

VIVIENNE: Don't you see he can't do his wonderful notes then. We're thinking of holding a dance in the playroom tonight. Eric's going to play on his mouth organ.

BARBARA: That awful noise.

ERIC: Women are heartless, aren't they, Doctor?

VIVIENNE: They can't be heartless because they've got hearts. I can feel mine beating. Have you listened to it with Doctor's stethoscope? It sounds like a train. [*They all listen. In putting back the stethoscope, they find a key.*]

ERIC: That's the key to the doctor's heart.

VIVIENNE: I've made a copy of it, and whenever I want something, I'll creep up quietly and open it. Doctor, were you ever a child?

DOCTOR: Yes, a long time ago.

VIVIENNE: What did it feel like? Did it feel funny to be small and thin with no hair on your face?

DOCTOR: I suppose I felt just like Eric feels now.

VIVIENNE: I don't believe you were ever small. You must have been born big.

ERIC: You've got to be small to be born. You can't come out otherwise. You girls know nothing.

BARBARA: What about Mary, she knows everything.

VIVIENNE: She thinks she's the cleverest in the world. She even says she's the best developed.

ERIC: I think she's the dirtiest. She says the most horrible things.

VIVIENNE: What about that new boy, William. The things he does in front of me. You wouldn't believe me if I told you, Doctor.

ERIC: Who's the best looking?

VIVIENNE: Barbara.

BARBARA: Julia.

VIVIENNE: Do you know John is Spanish? I wish I was. I would like to be an artist when I grow up. My Mum wants me to to be a stingy old dressmaker. All she thinks of is money.

ERIC: I wish I had some money. I'd give half of it to the doctor, and the other half I'd buy a regular mouth organ and penknife.

BARBARA: He'll soon grow up.

VIVIENNE: He's not as young as he used to be.

ERIC: Shall I tell you girls the story of the empty can?

BOTH: Do.

ERIC: There's nothing in it. [*Roars with laughter.*]

VIVIENNE: What big feet the doctor has! I wish I had big feet.

ERIC: You will when you grow older.

BARBARA: You just don't understand. She wants them now.

VIVIENNE: That's what my mother says whenever you ask her anything. 'You don't understand.'

BARBARA: Are you going to the cinema tomorrow, Eric?

ERIC: I think so. I can't remember having done anything naughty. But then you never can tell with nurses: they don't seem to allow for when you're ill. I feel a lot of electricity running through me in the morning and I get giddy. Then I feel giddy. But they never put me in the sick ward. Only girls go there.

BARBARA: Because girls are sicker than boys. Boys are strong. I think it's because girls are smaller.

ERIC: I felt pretty sick when I had laughing-gas to cut out my tonsils last time – didn't make me laugh, I can tell you. When I came round, there seemed to be a lot of children singing in my head. Before I went out – passed out – I saw a man go and get a penknife from the cupboard. I wouldn't have gone again for all the money in the world. When I saw the man go for the penknife, it made me sick in the stomach. Doctor, what would happen if you didn't pass any water? Geoffrey said you drown in it. I would hate that to happen to me. I s'pose they could always put in a syringe and take it out.

VIVIENNE: I'd never let them put a syringe into me.

ERIC: It couldn't happen to you. You haven't the same thing. It's only us.

VIVIENNE: I used to like Eric when I first came, but now I don't. I'm sure the doctor doesn't like you either.

ERIC: How d'you know?

VIVIENNE: I can feel it inside me. Isn't that so, Doctor?

DOCTOR: My own impression was I liked all of you.

ERIC: The doctors here always ask you whether you like your mother and father. How do they expect us to know that?

VIVIENNE: Sometimes I hate my Mum, and sometimes I like my Dad. And sometimes I hate both of them. Doctors ask you all sorts of silly questions – what you're going to be when you grow up. Every doctor I've met has asked me that.

ERIC: They probably try and find things out that way. I'd like to be a doctor when I grow up, but I haven't the brain.

VIVIENNE [*scornfully*]: You don't need brains. Look at the doctor. [*All laugh.*]

VIVIENNE [*to doctor*]: What are you supposed to be doing?

Group Psychotherapy

DOCTOR: My notes.

VIVIENNE: About us?

DOCTOR: No – I'm writing letters to the doctors of my other patients.

ERIC: Are they like us, or are they daft like Julia? [*a psychotic child*].

VIVIENNE [*laughing*]: You mean like you.

ERIC: Nurse B said tonight that once we left here you didn't bother about us any more. Is that true, Doctor?

DOCTOR: I don't quite know what Nurse B meant, but what you've just said is not true.

ERIC: Nurses shouldn't say that sort of thing because it's depressing for children. Nurse B has a cheek – she said that as I was going home you had finished with me.

VIVIENNE: I should hate anyone to say that of me. It makes me feel I'm not good enough.

BARBARA: Tonight we're going to play 'Consequences'. Will you play, Eric?

ERIC [*scornfully*]: I know. Vivienne is a nice girl, she loves John.

JOHN [*speaking for the first time*]: But she doesn't.

BARBARA [*looking admiringly at Eric's picture*]: Isn't his bird good?

VIVIENNE [*mockingly*]: Everything's good about Eric, I don't think. I wish someone would get my brother to come and help me. He's so funny. He always draws the same little man and he calls it Voss. I keep asking him to draw it, so one day he killed Voss and drew him dead with blood running out of his body. [*Barbara has been trying to make herself heard*] – I wonder what's she's saying?

BARBARA [*crossly*]: You're deaf.

VIVIENNE [*with dignity*]: I've been lots of things, but never deaf.

JOHN [*giggling*]: That's comical!

ERIC: When my Dad falls over anything and we all start laughing, he always says, 'Very comical.'

VIVIENNE: Do you laugh if he hurts himself?

ERIC: Not if he really hurts himself. We couldn't if he really hurts himself.

VIVIENNE: I laugh when my sister Gloria falls over.

BARBARA: I don't think it's fair to laugh if people fall down.

ERIC: I don't think it's funny when X twists my arm to get me down the stairs.

VIVIENNE: X once beat me on the behind all the way down the stairs.

ERIC: I don't think it's nice to hit a girl on her behind, do you, Doctor?

DOCTOR: Why isn't it nice, Eric?

ERIC: Because girls are different from boys. You can hit boys on the behind.

VIVIENNE: I don't see the difference, but it's nice of you to say so, Eric.

ERIC [*doggedly*]: Well, I wouldn't do it myself.

BARBARA [*laughing*]: Eric thinks we have softer behinds.

ERIC: Well, it's true. That's why girls don't play football – they might be hit behind.

VIVIENNE: What nonsense, Eric.

ERIC: Girls are not as strong as boys. Just look at Mary. [*They all laugh.*]

BARBARA: She's dying!

VIVIENNE: Yes, she's dying.

ERIC: She thinks she's very ill.

VIVIENNE: She says her temperature is 104.

BARBARA: She tries to make out that she's ill. [*Proudly*] I had a temperature of 100. Ain't that a lot, Vivienne?

VIVIENNE [*unkindly*]: You don't half talk bad language – 'ain't'! No one will marry you if you talk like that.

BARBARA: Are you going to get married, Vivienne? [*John leaves the room to go to the lavatory.*]

VIVIENNE: I've got to be, because I want babies to wash and dress. I'd like teeny-weeny ones, the size of a thimble.

ERIC [*laughing*]: You can have them that size without getting married.

BARBARA: Will you get married, Eric?

ERIC: It's not a question of getting married. It's who's going to marry me. It's very easy just to say 'get married'. You've got to find a nice girl.

VIVIENNE: So girls are some use after all. Boys make out they're everything. Nurse said when my comb fell down into a lavatory-pan, 'Go and get a boy to take it out.' I hadn't thought of that. I must say it was a good idea.

ERIC: J threw my shoe into the lavatory-pan. He throws everything into the lavatory-pan.

BARBARA: I'd like to throw him into the lavatory-pan.

ERIC [*laughing*]: That's a good one. Doctor, tell me this. What's the difference between me and an elephant?

DOCTOR: Well, the elephant's got four legs and a trunk, for instance.

ERIC: No. I mean the *real* difference.

DOCTOR: I don't know. You tell me.

ERIC [*triumphantly*]: You hear him everyone. He doesn't know the difference between us and elephants. We can't trust him to be our doctor.

THE OTHERS [*laughing*]: No, we can't.

VIVIENNE: I told you the best place for him is his coffin. Then I would take his place and be the doctor.

ERIC: No, it would have to be me. It has to be a man.

VIVIENNE [*scornfully*]: You're not a man. I'm as much a man as you are.

ERIC [*laughing*]: Oh, no you're not. Can she be, Doctor? She can't.
VIVIENNE: You don't shave.
ERIC: I will one day; you never will. Put that in your hat and eat it.
BARBARA [*to Vivienne*]: He's just showing off.
JOHN [*suddenly*]: I'd like to be doctor.
ALL [*laughing*]: Imagine John!
ERIC: I expect you've got to be awfully clever first.
VIVIENNE: What's clever in sitting and talking? That's all he does.
ERIC: He's got to look at your tonsils sometimes. Doctor, do girls have tonsils?
VIVIENNE: Of course they have, stupid.
ERIC: I heard only boys had tonsils. Girls were born without any. [*Vivienne and Barbara both open their mouths.*]
VIVIENNE: Look and see what big ones I've got. They want to cut them out, but I'm not going to let them.
BARBARA [*complacently*]: We've got everything only boys don't know it. Boys always show off for nothing.

What is most noticeable in these extracts is the unobtrusive participation of the therapist in the group. He makes comments, he asks questions, he is playful and colloquial. There is very little direct interpretation and then only in somewhat general terms, for example, 'The dream may simply mean that you have some worries about growing up and that you probably feel that you're not going to make much of a showing.' The anxiety and tension is deliberately kept at a fairly low level, and the group often seems to be enjoying the session. There is no opening up of the more negative and hostile feelings for the therapist–adult.

Within the last seven years, the group-analytic approach to the latency child has become much more verbal, analytic, and interpretative, with a focus on the positive and negative aspects of the group but not the individual relationship with the therapist. The activity period has been done away with altogether in favour of a single-phase group session in which the activity occurred spontaneously and was then a matter for discussion. Interpretations, from the beginning, were liberal and were directed at the group. Development was spontaneous, without programme or occupation, and the members were confronted with their own tensions, anxieties, and silences. The early interpretations were pointed towards the affective upheavals of initiation, and were designed to create an environment of increasing psychological awareness. Every comment, however trivial, peripheral, and irrelevant, was purposefully exploited in this manner, and it was not infrequent for the group to react with exasperation at the way in which the therapist referred everything almost automatically back to the here and now of the therapeutic situation. The first sessions were primarily used to inculcate this sort of orientation, and prepared the way for later interpretations of process and content. These, when inspected serially, gave the impression of remarkable consistency because, no matter what the content emerging in the situation, it was transposed into the context of a group response to the therapist. Many of these early interpretations were nothing better than broad analogies between external events and group events and between past events and present ones occurring in the treatment milieu. Having phenomena 'manipulated' in this way 'before their very eyes' made the group understandably suspicious, and it was important for the therapist to get across to the patients that he recognized and appreciated the reasons for their mistrustfulness, since they were not to know as yet how closed the group-analytic situation was and how immune the therapist was to parental encroachments or pressures. Finally, they still could not know what to expect from the therapy. It was also imperative for the therapist to make it as clear as he could that the group was meeting for treatment purposes and that the members were there to deal with each other's problems. It was not up to him to lay down how the group was to go about its therapeutic business; he wisely allowed them to find this out for themselves.

Perhaps the most characteristic thing about this second latency technique were the conditions under which it was practised. The disadvantage of working with children of this age group in a large room gradually became clearer over the years. The large room allowed the children to scatter, to get away from the therapist, to become inaccessible to interpretations, and to become caught up in fragmented group activities and sub-group formations. The idea of the small room evolved from the need to keep the members in close therapeutic contact with the therapist. The room is bare and has no furniture except a small table and a set of chairs. Six active children plus the therapist seem to fill it to capacity and at times to make it feel like the Black Hole of Calcutta. The original room used for this purpose was no more than six by twelve feet, and the children had to squeeze past the therapist's chair to get around the room.

Group Psychotherapy

There is only one explicit rule to this group situation, which is that there is 'no exit'. As in the Sartre play *In Camera,** everyone is in it together, and everyone has to continue together however small the room may appear to become, and however tense and uncomfortable the situation may grow. There is no doubt that the atmosphere can be 'hellish' at times especially during the early stages, and a considerable amount of noise and aggression can be generated. This is, again, a form of contract which the children learn to respect, so much so that even when a child wants to go to the toilet, a great deal of group discussion can take place because everyone wants to know what 'exactly' he is up to. It can be treated as a joke and can also become a serious matter of protocol. As long as the therapist is there to share everything with the group and the group is there to share everything with the therapist, and the group life is preserved within the four walls of the small room, the rapidity of the therapeutic progress is often astonishing.

With boys, the implicit suggestion to sit and talk seems to strike at the very roots of their masculine anxieties. Coming close together or being passive and verbal is tantamount to being sissy, and interpretations relating to closeness or distance often have an immediate and profound effect on the group, scattering it to the far corners of the room, involving it in fights, or bringing it anxiously to within arm's reach of the therapist. There is, thus, a constant centripetal centrifugal movement of the group as a whole in relation to the therapist. During the early sessions, when the children first discover the opportunity afforded them to express themselves, the level of noise can be considerable. Interpretations are apparently 'lost' within the maelstrom. Later, at quieter moments, they come back from the group, having been heard. Experience shows that little that the therapist says goes unperceived. He does not need to shout or chase after the children. They are much too aware of him and hyper-alerted to his voice and expression. To a great extent he enjoys a relative diplomatic immunity from flying objects, and the less anxious or concerned he is about being hurt, the less likely is he to be hit.

The therapist's initial comments deal with the natural anxieties of a strange situation and the expectable suspiciousness provoked by a strange individual. Next, he anticipates perplexities and misconceptions to do with the treatment process. After about the

* See page 133.

tenth session, his interpretations veer around to the relationship between the group and the therapist, their closeness or distance from him, and the underlying significance of the therapeutic encounter. The special psychological environment having been created, the children, with surprising rapidity, begin to think in psychological terms and to search for the latent behind the manifest content. By about the twentieth session, the group will begin to make direct interpretations towards one another, and the therapist now reserves his own interpretations for those moments when the members come together for the implicit purpose of attacking, defeating, seducing, and escaping from him. By 'shutting in' the group, constructing a sensitive situation and interpreting the group-therapist relationship actively, the effectiveness of the treatment condition is much enhanced.

The early phases of the group with girls is not too dissimilar. The same techniques apply, but the behaviour of the participants is somewhat different. The girls are much more likely to express themselves through passivity, silence, shyness, and nervous interaction, characterized by giggling and whispered communication. They develop the same anxiety and anger over the unstructured nature of the group meetings and its apparent pointlessness, but their exasperations are expressed much more in verbal terms. With a male therapist in the girls' group, the members are immediately confronted with the problems of sex difference and age difference. The heterosexual dangers come to the forefront in much the same way as the homosexual crises that arise in the boy's group. Girls, in general, show greater skill in dissipating tension than do the boys, who are more given to 'acting out' their disturbances.

The following is an illustration of a first session with a group of prepubertal boys, using the active technique.

The children are obviously anxious, insecure, and constrained, and Dr M, the therapist, comments that since they don't know each other, perhaps it might be helpful if they introduced themselves to one another. This is done, after which the group falls silent again. Dr M comments that perhaps all of them are thinking that they don't know what they are there for. At this, one of the boys turns to the therapist and asks what the treatment was about. The therapist turns the question back to the boys, but they look bewildered and shake their heads. The therapist remarks that it sounds as though they want to hear about this from him. There is general agreement. He then proceeds to tell them, simply and directly, that he himself sees the situation as one where they can talk about anything; he understands that they have many concerns and that they are finding it hard to share these with other people or bring them out in the open; but they are all here to talk about such things and to get to know one another better and also themselves. Silence again falls, and after it has gone on for a short period, the therapist reflects that one of the things they would be doing in the group together would be trying to understand what they were doing in the group together, and he wonders what it means that they are all so quiet. This is followed by another period of silence. One of the boys begins picking at the surface of the table in a somewhat strained manner, and another remarks (and it is the first spontaneous remark of the session) that if he continues doing this, there soon won't be any table left at all. As the boys smile at this, the therapist tells them that he hopes their smiling means that they are aware of the many things a fellow did when he got nervous or anxious, and that picking at the table could be one of them. The scratching immediately stops, and the boy who has made the first 'interpretation' wants to know what the mothers were doing together in the room upstairs. (They are holding a concurrent group session.) The therapist wonders what the boys think about this but obtains no comments. After the next silence, the therapist remarks that each of the boys had earlier introduced himself but that he had not introduced himself and that perhaps some of their silence was related to their questions about him, what he was, and why he was there. The children immediately nod their agreement, so the therapist goes on to say a few words about himself in terms of being interested in problems and wanting to help about them.

At the end of his statement, one of the boys takes out a bunch of firecrackers from his pocket which are closely inspected and lead to a general discussion about fireworks in terms of their explosive and dangerous qualities. From this the conversation shifts to cigarette smoking, and mention is made of some 'neat guys' who have been smoking on the quiet outside their homes, and have gotten into trouble. When the expression 'gotten into trouble' is made, the therapist picks this up and remarks that the boys might well be concerned about whether they would get into trouble if they let out their secrets in the group. They must surely worry what the therapist would do about it, especially whether he would tell their mothers. The boys immediately pounce on this, admitting that it had concerned them, and wondering, in fact, just what the therapist would do with all the information they gave him. The therapist deems it important at this point to make an 'official' statement concerning confidentiality and of the necessity to keep everything that took place in the room within the room.

The group interpretations in this first session were, therefore, directed towards the initial nervousness about the treatment situation, at the imagined dangerousness of what might happen, and at the mistrust of the therapist as another adult who might 'tell on them' and get them into further trouble. There was also a special reference to the meaning of silence in a group setting. What the therapist was, therefore, engaged in doing throughout the session was constructing a treatment model to serve the group for the direction of the treatment. The children were being oriented towards the group situation as a specialized treatment environment, towards themselves as people with problems, and towards the therapist as someone who was concerned with understanding the nature of their problems. This was sufficient group work for a first session.

As a contrast, we can take a briefer look at a first session in a girl's group.

Once again, the initial introductions are followed by the same sort of embarrassed silence, but the girls in a more socially skilful way manage to steer the conversation into a neutral topic. The therapist, as usual, waits for a suitable opening and then begins to wonder aloud, now that everybody knows who everybody else is, what they are going to do with each other and with their time. This, predictably, introduces an immediate silence. The girls are conscious that the manner in which the therapist has cut into the 'tea-party talk' clearly indicates that he is not terribly interested in that quality of interchange, and so they find themselves without their habitual resource. During the silence, they shift about restlessly and sigh, and the therapist again wonders aloud who is going to break the ice, beside himself. He points out that people who come into a group like this for the first time must surely have a lot of questions about it – about each other and, more especially, about the therapist. After another painful silence, one of the girls makes an effort to put matters on a more tolerable plane of anxiety and begins talking about her school's new swimming-pool and of how one of the girls, who was a non-swimmer, had jumped in at the deep end. The therapist immediately intervenes to remark that that is rather like the situation here. They are all wondering who is going to jump in first, and what the dangers are. None of them had been in this sort of situation before, and so would be unable to know where it is shallow and where it is deep. As far as this is concerned, they are all non-swimmers. The group are startled by the twist in the conversation and the therapist adds a further mysterious comment: 'I suppose you are all wondering just what I am getting at. It is hard,' he says, 'to get into a situation like group therapy (and he deliberately uses the term 'group therapy') where you meet a bunch of new people that you have never seen before. You just don't know what to say. You want to know something about it, but you don't know how to even ask. I am sure you all want me to say just why we are all meeting here.' One of the girls takes this up: 'It would certainly help if you would say why everybody's here,' to which the therapist replies: 'Well, we're here to talk about whatever comes into our minds to see if we can use our thoughts to understand ourselves better, and especially to understand why we are here and why we feel so uncomfortable about being here.' 'Everybody is scared,' says one of the girls, 'that they might say something wrong.' The therapist immediately agrees that this could be a big problem. It isn't so easy to say what one is thinking about, especially if one doesn't know the other people and what it is going to be used for. Another girl mentions that she always feels very shy about talking, but that she might as well jump into the water first. There is general laughter about this which seems to relieve the general anxiety. Taking courage from this, the girl goes on to say that she has a little puppy at home that eats at the table and spits when you feed it. The therapist remarks: 'Maybe it's frightened. Like everybody here is a little frightened.' Again there is a slightly embarrassed laugh from the group. After a while someone asks: 'Why don't we just sit around the table?' to which the therapist answers: 'We can do this any way you like,' and again there is silence for a while. Another of the children begins talking about school and what fun they have fooling around during recess. Once again the therapist refers the matter back to the group situation and remarks: 'I suppose everybody must be wondering if we can fool around here in the same way.' No matter what the children say in relation to the world outside, the group therapist brings them back to the group situation, and they begin to notice this. Soon it becames a reference point for the girls themselves, and when this happens, it indicates that the group is really launched.

The first session is, in many respects, the key session in group therapy. The group members are taught to look at the group through the eyes of the group therapist, and, as it begins, so it will go. They learn a little about groups, a little about therapy, something about the therapeutic process, something about the role of the therapist, and something about the therapist's expectations with regard to his patients. It, almost inevitably, follows the same course of introductions, awkwardness, silences, growing effects, releases of tension, covering up defences, anxious mistrustfulness, descent into trivialities, group interpretations, reference back to the group situation, interpretations of concern regarding the therapist, and problems of confidentiality.

If used consistently, this technique of bringing everything back to the group situation, and of consistently interpreting the group response to the therapist, gradually leads to a series of developments. A first phase is one of defensive pandemonium which the group has to work through and the therapist has to live through, and live through it he must if he is to move on to the next phase. In the second phase, the amount of movement, aggression, and noise is reduced considerably. The boys actually sit around for periods and begin to examine highly charged emotional material brought in from the outside or generated within the group situation. In the third phase, the insight of the group is at its height, and the group begins to interpret its own behaviour so that less use is made of the therapist in this connexion. The ultimate conflict between the therapist and the group in the boys' group involves their image of him as the archetypal disciplinarian, from whom all punishment stems and with whom peace must eventually be made if the individual is to survive in the group. The therapeutic experience was perceived as a demasculinizing demand on the active, aggressive boy, and required to be resisted to the end. Surrender in the girls' group signified the emergence of active, angry, envious wishes cloaked for the most part by passive, erotic insinuation and preoccupations. In both instances rage against the therapist represented the necessary intermediate experience. An example of the problems involved in externalizing the nuclear conflicts follows.

4. ILLUSTRATION FROM THE TWENTY-FIRST SESSION OF A BOYS' GROUP

All the boys are here today, and they come in immediately and start talking about their summer holidays that are pending. Since the therapist is going on vacation, there is also a good deal of talk about this, especially in terms of getting rid of him and doing without him. The boys then begin to play actively with a catapult, shooting clay out of the window, and some of them turn the chairs over in the room. The therapist points out that they all seem to be trying to show how strong and active and masculine they are. At this point one of the boys becomes frantically aggressive, and the therapist picks up on this and reminds the group of a story that this boy had once told them about another boy in his school who always felt very weak and inadequate and so he had to act particularly tough. At this, the boy proceeds to grab a lighter and make as if to set fire to the chair, and another group member laughingly comments that he must have got awfully angry at the therapist's comment. This reduces the fire setter to a state of extreme sullenness and disgust, but the other members of the group are quite startled by the interpretation. The therapist remarks to the group that a person who is worried about himself and his feelings often needs to act in precisely this way, and it is the function of the group to understand this need. He appreciates that they have done so. At this, in a very organized fashion, all the boys proceed methodically and systematically to turn every bit of furniture in the room upside down. Once they have done so, they sit around on the upside-down table and chairs and talk for the next forty minutes in a very free and open fashion devoid of any hurly-burly behaviour. The fire setter begins by discussing a situation at home that morning when he had become intensely angry with his mother. This draws from another member the envious, admiring comment that this is something he would never be able to do. Each of the boys then in turn mention instances of sudden, extreme anger with their mothers, which they delineate with much feeling. At the height of the catharsis, one of the boys tells a story he had seen on television. It concerns a man who is sitting at a table with another man who notices his somewhat ornate cigarette lighter. The first man then offers to make a sporting bet with him. He would hand him over his brand new convertible car if he could operate the lighter successfully ten times in succession. If he fails, he has to sacrifice one of his fingers. The bet is made, and they then repair to a hotel room where the second man proceeds to light the lighter eight times in a row, and as he goes on to the ninth trial, the first man's wife comes in and says: 'Thank God, I've come in time,' and describes how her husband has been banished from his first country after collecting forty-seven fingers and losing eleven cars, and how, finally, she had managed to restrain this by winning from him all his possessions, so that he was unable to engage in any further bets. At this moment she reaches down to pick up the lighter with a fingerless hand!

As he finishes telling the story, there is a stunned silence around the room, and the therapist points out how anxious the story has made all the boys, and wonders whether there isn't something in it that reflects what they have all been struggling with for a long time in the group. There is no direct response to this, but the boys, almost tangentially, begin a series of interchanges around jokes and riddles. After about ten minutes of this, the therapist remarks quietly that something has struck him rather forcibly, and he is curious whether anybody has any idea what it is. (This enigmatic way of presenting an interpretation is usually very effective in latency groups.) The boys eagerly speculate about it, one suggesting that it has to do with the fact that they had split up into different sub-groups, another, that they have been avoid ing something, etc. The speculations are mostly about things that they are not doing. Finally, the therapist intervenes with the comment that what in fact had struck him had been that they had taken the room and turned it completely upside down, and had then been sitting around and talking for over half an hour, and he raises the question as to whether what they are saying through this is that it is impossible to sit around and talk in the ordinary way because it makes them feel weak and girlish, that is, missing in something just as girls are. (The boys have frequently been curious as to what girls do in a group like this, feeling sure it is different from what they themselves do.) Therefore, the therapist goes on, in order to be able to function like girls and not become girls, they have first to turn everything upside down. Only in an upside-down world can they dare to behave in that way.

There is a long silence after this comment. Eventually one of the boys looks up at the therapist and wants to know what kind of cigarette he smokes. The therapist asks what he has in mind. There is no direct response to this, but the boys then talk about the things you put in people's cigarettes that make them blow up. The therapist wonders aloud if the boys aren't reflecting a wish in relation to him, and they all laugh at this and joke about it. In their 'collective phantasy' they imagine getting hold of his cigarette and filling it with some substance which when lit would create a tremendous smell! The therapist remarks humorously that they certainly are paying him back in kind for his ideas about boys and girls and the fears they have about 'missing' something in the situation. Soon after this, the boy who had started the upside-down movement now goes to the various pieces of furniture and begins constructively to turn them right side up again with the help of other members in the group. They ask who is going to clean up the room, and express a great deal of concern about this. The therapist remarks that they seem to be feeling guilty about the feelings they have had about him during the session and are now wanting to wipe out any evidence of what has gone on in the room, and make amends for it. The interpretation beings about an explosive departure of the boys from the room.

In the girls' group, as in the boys' group, the members are very much concerned about their feelings for the therapist. This gets displaced on to accounts of innocent heterosexual experiences, about the tricks that bigger boys play on them, about being teased and tormented by brothers and fathers, about growing up and being accepted, and about having an attractive appearance. At times they would punitively exclude the therapist from 'their' groups as being contitutionally incapable of understanding what little girls think about. At other times they secretively and seductively focus on some feminine object such as a handbag over which they laugh and giggle with regard to contents which on no account can be shown to a man. Much of this leads quite logically and inevitably into concerns about their fathers, who are frequently described as being 'too nosey' about their daughters. Girls, on the whole, are more likely to deal with transference resistances by wanting to give up therapy or withdrawing totally from further discussion, so that the group at its most resistant is also at its quietest. The 'small room' never feels overwhelmingly small. One has only to watch the two kinds of groups to realize why boys always outnumber girls in clinic referrals. The latter's disturbances so much less obtrusive or obnoxious.

The two modes of approach that have been discussed with regard to latency children are in principle the same, but vary in the intensity of the group situation created and in the activity of the group therapist. Both types are verbal and analytic, but the operational level of anxiety is kept down to a minimum in the first kind, which is suitable for the mildly to moderately neurotic child with a largely internalized conflict and a good deal of superimposed inhibition. The second approach is especially effective with the more acting-out, pre-delinquent, or delinquent type of child who has to become more neurotic before he can be treated effectively by psychotherapy, that is, his tendency to activity must give place to the need to verbalize. This latter variety is undoubtedly more exacting to handle and less comfortable to live through. It requires, on the whole, more group experience, since the transformation from acting out to speaking out is technically a difficult matter. This kind of defensiveness is a problem in individual psychotherapy, and, when summated in the group situation, it can lead to concerted aggression or avoidance that can ultimately defeat the analytic process unless the therapist relentlessly persists in pursuing his 'internalizing' technique. In the process of being converted from an asocial into a neurotic group, the 'gang' becomes a 'group', and the group formations change from socially derived structures to predominantly neurotic ones.

The group members eventually come to see group therapy through the eyes of the group analyst. They come to regard it as an important, serious event in their daily lives, to be missed only under conditions that require lengthy explanations, not rationalizations, to the group. Absences are, therefore, rare events in these analytically oriented sessions. As always, the essence of good group therapy is to know your group, more particularly the tension level at which it functions best, and to know yourself, your tolerance for tension-inducing behaviour, and for the positive and negative feelings aroused in you by the sustained pressures of the children.

5. THE 'SMALL CIRCLE' TECHNIQUE WITH ADOLESCENT GROUPS

Adolescent groups are best conducted in a bare, non-distracting room with comfortable chairs arranged in a fairly small circle, smaller than the adult circle, so that physical contact is never very far away. As in all analytic-type groups, the members are faced with a non-structured situation by which, characteristically, they are at first perplexed and then made resentful and angry. Once again the therapist confines himself initially to comments on the group feelings and behaviour, and once again the outside world is brought inside to the group situation, so that it gradually becomes the ultimate framework of reference for all types of material introduced by the members. As time goes on, the group gradually becomes aware of the therapist's consistent practice – that he invariably searches for the latent behind the manifest intent, and that he is always envisaging the group as a whole, however individually their problems present themselves.

The circle, as with the adult groups, is empty so that nothing intervenes between the members, and there is nothing to hide behind. Under conditions of stress, the group often spontaneously and unconsciously contracts or expands the circle depending on the nature of the current anxieties. The regressive–progressive movement described in the section on phenomenology is especially characteristic of adolescent groups and requires a high degree of flexibility on the part of the therapist. At times he may find himself dealing with mature viewpoints and adult topics, when, all of a sudden, he is confronted with an acute regression and a primitive response that seems utterly out of keeping with the situation he has been dealing with. The therapist must mainly concern himself with the interpretative recognition of the group movement, whether progressive or regressive, and the group dynamics that have initiated them. If he treats them at their face value, the group will accuse him of misunderstanding them.

Questions of identity become increasingly important during the course of therapy, both in relation to personal identities, as well as in relation to the group identity (the 'collective image'), and to their growing awareness of the identity of the therapist and his capacity for stimulating the ideals of the group. In this context, he is regarded as one who has coped successfully with maturation, and as such, is both an object of respect and a representative of reality.

On other occasions he is seen in the contrasting image of the regressive seducer, tempting them back into childhood with all its parental-oriented attractions and dependencies. He is no longer a new figure with whom they want to identify but an old figure whom they want to be rid of, and as the group oscillates between one position and the other, the therapist is pushed one way or the other, or, to put it more accurately, he follows in one direction or the other depending on the needs of the group.

The mixed adolescent group appears to be too disturbing or too inhibiting for most adolescent patients, and so it has become fairly general practice to keep them to the one sex. The optimal number is about six. Beyond this figure the group becomes more difficult to control, and excessive 'acting out' and sub-grouping may occur. The members themselves usually prefer a group of five to six.

The sex of the therapist makes an appreciable difference to the group reaction, bringing out the two aspects of the central adolescent problem. A male therapist in a girls' group gets a lot of positive father transference from the more mature type of girl, but is treated with resentment or indifference by the immature one. The female therapist may have to cope with much hostility from the maturer girl and a demanding dependency from the immature. The reverse is true for the boys' group, but the older more mature boy may find the female therapist 'too sissy' for his needs and will turn to the male therapist for his identification patterns and ideals. Similarly, a well groomed, self-sufficient young woman may stimulate identifications more than rivalries and 'mother' reactions. The tolerance of the therapist is put to a stern test, especially earlier on, but if he can survive the repeated crises that punctuate the progress of the group, he will find the experience among the more rewarding in the field of group work.

The so-called adolescent 'crises' are seen in 'pure culture' in the adolescent group. The twin problems of coming to final satisfactory terms with the past, and facing the mature tasks of the future, fill the present with uncertainty, especially in those whose upbringing has been neglectful or over-protected. Adolescence has been called 'a state of suspension', and in the group situation one can sometimes observe the way in which the intense conflict ensuing from the opposing attractions of the past and future, between the regressive and progressive forces, and between the homosexual and heterosexual tendencies, lead to an apathetic disregard of everything but the passing moment.

The language of early adolescence is still hyperbolical. Interchanges are rapid with some inclination to oratory. The all-pervasive fear is of sounding 'phoney'. Silences are alarming, especially in girls' groups, when whispering between pairs may relieve the tension. 'Secrets' from the conductor are much relished, again, more especially in girls' groups.

Among the specific group factors, 'mirror reactions' are constant, and both positive and negative effects are highly contagious. Members passing through a negative phase may combine together against the therapist. Such concerted hostility is greater if there is a preponderance of rebellion-minded delinquents. The group, as one might expect, remains leader-centred for a much longer time than is the case in adult groups.

The regressive and progressive 'movements' in the group need to be carefully watched. Treating the members as potentially mature adults, with the right to regress on some occasions, helps in the handling of both 'movements'. Too much should not be expected nor disappointment shown when the group fails to live up to expectations. The aspirations of the group therapist may occasionally be too much for the group.

Thematic developments show little consistency or coherence in their evolution. 'Crushes' within the group are a popular topic, but 'sucking up' to the conductor is strongly condemned. Childhood is often discussed nostalgically, and the future with a certain amount of trepidation. As the group matures, progressive topics such as marriage, employment, hobbies, etc, become more frequent. Strong transference attachments provoke jealousy reactions. For girls, menstruation is a stock theme, and many strange theories are woven around its occurrence. For boys, involuntary seminal emissions at night may bring into focus many unusual fears. Dreams are a favourite preoccupation for both sexes, and wild interpretations and even wilder 'associations' are lavishly offered. Group dreams are more frequent than in adult groups. These dreams give a dynamic indication of the relational state; members are excluded or included on a simple wish-fulfilling principle. Magical thinking is frequent and takes the form of superstitious rituals with respect to the group circle.

Illustration from an adolescent group (*girls*). Ages: 14–16. Symptom Group: Anxiety hysteria. Numbers: 6. Session 15.

This short record is interesting as it shows the sudden sharp regressive swing away from a progressive movement dealing with future marital, housing, and nursery plans, with special emphasis on baby rearing. It also illustrates how the mood of an adolescent group, more especially of girls, tends to swing as a whole. Social imitation, empathy, and sympathy seem to be at their height with this age group.

B: We don't think we'll talk about babies today. We're fed up of babies. We're sick of babies. We think they're dirty.

J: I'm never going to have one and I don't care who knows it. I'd much rather have a kitten. They're nice and soft. Babies are hard like meat.

B: They stink! I wouldn't have one near me for anything.

F: I think it's a cheek asking us to have them. It's all because of you that we have them [*looking at the doctor*]. [*Everyone giggles at this and F blushes.*] Well, you get them born or something. I mean doctors.

J: Kittens can sit cosy in front of a nice fire. No one's cruel to kittens. I wish V would stop giggling and say something.

V: I think babies have the best time. They drown kittens. I want to be a baby – but I should like to know it's me. [*Getting excited*] I know, I could have my own brain and be inside a baby's body, then I should have such a nice time.

DOCTOR: But someone would need to have the babies to provide you with the bodies.

V [*slowly*]: I never thought of that. I suppose babies can't have babies.

In the previous session, it was the same 'mass' response to the progressive feelings. The adolescents react from session to session as if they were constantly confronted by this great question of choice and with it the attendant fear of committing themselves permanently. They look upon the therapist as a committed person and question him about his choice; why did he become a doctor, get married, have children? Didn't he realize he would have to die one day? All people who allow themselves to grow up face the prospect of death....

The group-analytic adolescent group provides one of the best preparations for maturity.

6. GROUP THERAPEUTIC TECHNIQUES FOR RESIDENTIAL UNITS

In a residential treatment centre or in-patient ward setting, the institution can be structured along group lines. Such group organizations may include children's groups, staff groups, combined groups of staff and children, and parent groups. This deployment of interlocking groups has certain important advantages for institutional life. In the first place, it gives everyone, staff included, the experience of the same therapeutic environment. It therefore cuts across such tension-creating dichotomies as staff and patient, adult and child, treater and treated, superior and inferior, and most important, 'us' and 'them'. It reduces the hierarchical discontinuities and the authoritarian procedures that stem from them. If all the staff are included in the organization, then the child begins to see that the adult who serves their meals or washes their pants or gossips to them in the kitchen can be just as helpful, in their own way, as the adult who teaches them in school, sounds their chest with the stethoscope, or talks to them in private interviews. The whole range of helpfulness of the institution comes into better perspective and, as in the case of the extended family group, the child does not put too many of his emotional eggs in one basket. He becomes increasingly discriminating in his use of the help available and knows whom to go to with what. This is an important life attitude to cultivate in the child since one of the basic problems of many adult patients is that they so often get to the wrong doctors and are, therefore, treated for the wrong things. It eventually may take many failures and disappointments to reach the right therapist for their condition.

The other valuable use of group organization is the early location of disturbances so that they no longer occur suddenly, unexpectedly, and catastrophically. The covert life of a community can be brought into the open, and the 'collective unconscious' with its troublesome mysteries of devils and angels, gives place to a rational collective consciousness. The institution organized on group lines establishes, as it were, a number of radar machines located at different strategic points, so that even minimal disturbances can be easily picked up. The same staff member can be participating in the children's group, in the staff–children's group, in the staff group, and in the parent–staff group, so that if any section of the community is disturbed by personal or interpersonal difficulties, it soon becomes evident just where the disturbance is located, at what level it is operating, and what is its nature, intensity, and pattern. By pattern is meant the dynamic interpersonal configuration or more concretely the number of personnel interlocked at any one time in conflict. What has been called a *configurational analysis* in group therapy involves determining the nature and extent of the interaction and the location of the centre of the disturbance.

The groups composed of staff and children are as difficult to handle as family groups. The staff may have grave doubts about it and are often concerned about losing face, especially in front of their colleagues, and the children inevitably feel outnumbered and at the usual child-to-adult disadvantage. In this type of group, the grievances of the children and the counter grievances of the staff are made centres of discussion. Complaints can become positive contributions if they are treated in reciprocal fashion – that is, in a two-way process with bilateral systems of respect and understanding at work. The children need to understand the difficulties of the staff in handling collections of children, and the staff have to learn to appreciate the many and varied problems of group-upbringing. Honesty and straightforwardness are essential to the functioning of this type of group. In one such situation, a little girl remarked: 'Don't you sometimes feel that you would like to give us all a good bashing. If I were you, I would want to or else I would explode. It must be awful to keep it all inside you.' The immediate response to the girl's remarks was a series of defences put forward by the staff members against the suggestion that the staff could have negative feelings *at all*. They were there, they said, for the good of the children. Because of their completely adult status and maturity, and because of their enormous professional permissiveness and tolerance, their only reaction lay in the direction of greater understanding of the children. 'We are here to understand you,' said one, 'that's our job. If we were to become cross, we should fail in our jobs.' The jobs, it appeared, gave them this superhuman ability not to feel the daily pricks and arrows of outrageous children. There was no room for counter-action and counter-feeling. The child who made the statement clearly assumed that the staff felt the same as she did but simply concealed it better. 'If I were you,' she seemed to be saying, 'I would feel cross, so where has the crossness gone?' And that was certainly the key question: Where *had* the crossness gone? The group leader agreed with the children that it must have gone *somewhere*; had the staff become more tense? More anxious? More persecuted? More negativistic? More pompous? Had they kicked the institution's cat? Or developed migraine? Abdominal pain? Or pains in the neck?

Such defence mechanisms against sexual and aggressive feelings towards the children can be obliquely dealt with in the staff groups much better than in the groups made up of children and staff. The staff groups should be run by an outsider with no emotional axe to grind for himself and with a reasonable degree of non-involvement in the maelstrom of institutional life.

In such a setting, the matter of counter-feelings can be approached by discussing certain basic assumptions. First of all, it was generally the case that people who take up child-caring work with children have unconscious reasons for it which often relate to their own childhood and parent–child relationships. They may be motivated, therefore, by the need to undo some dreadful misunderstanding of the past, by the need to identify with certain disturbances in children similar to what they had manifested themselves in childhood, by the need to express certain unsatisfied feelings and impulses towards brothers and sisters, or by the overriding compulsion to rescue children from predicaments that had once been a source of injury and suffering to themselves. It was, therefore, imperative to look at one's motives for child work when one encountered difficulties with children.

Secondly, there was nothing intrinsically wrong with feelings, even socially unacceptable feelings, provided we learned how to recognize them and handle them. When these remained largely unconscious, they could be used, in hysterical fashion, to identify too closely with the children, or, in obsessional fashion, to release sadistic and masochistic wishes with the help of certain rigidities and routines, or in paranoid fashion, to make monsters and victims of certain children, or, if the defences were less than satisfactory, to live in a constant haze of anxious apprehension. Even a superficial analysis of these defending and attacking mechanisms – the mechanisms of attack are as many and as varied and as disguised as the mechanisms of defence – can lead to an opening up of conflicts. In any group, there is usually a mixed assortment of attackers and defenders, the attackers attacking and not aware that they are attacking or trying to conceal their intentions or even denying it; the defenders defending and not knowing that they are defending and denying that they have anything to be defensive about. Confronting the group with its naked intentions is one of the factors that can lead to the disruption of the group, but the truth in therapy need never be made too suddenly or too shockingly. In these quasi-therapeutic situations, it is well to bear in mind the well-known political course of *gradualism.* All these matters can be learned deeply and meaningfully and slowly. Since Freud, no one has ever been in a hurry with psychotherapy. The key word in this context has always been 'interminable'.

The third assumption is that there is a need to give and take in all human relationships. Sometimes we give too much and feel resentful, or take too much and feel greedy, but, in general, most of us enjoy both roles. Whenever we come to deal with patients or children, some of us begin to think that we have only to give and no longer take. It is true that maladjusted children can be exceedingly demanding, and drain us of our feeling with parasitic pleasure, giving little or nothing back in return, but no unilateral relationship in human society is a good one. It may be better to give than to receive, but unilateral giving is bad for both sides. It is always therapeutically wise to expect something in return, even from the most psychotic child, for whom the act of giving may become the act of redemption. Any human being who allows himself to be constantly treated as a cupboard will, eventually, find it as bare as that of Mother Hubbard. He has a duty to himself to replenish his stores of love from time to time.

Many caretakers of children believe it to be their official purpose to drain themselves of feeling for the sake of the children, like some self-sacrificing mothers. They see themselves as givers, asking nothing in return, and this is what they consider so admirably therapeutic – that their loving is unconditional. Such an attitude, on analysis, frequently reveals itself as a defence against an inner feeling of greed. They have to do something for nothing because they want everything. In the group, no attempt is made to analyse such primitive reactions, but their existence can be profitably pointed out. It should be shown:

(1) That unilateral receiving is not therapeutic for the child.

(2) That unilateral giving is not healthy for the adult.

(3) That the establishment of a reciprocal relationship is as good an ending-point to short-term therapy as any.

(4) That the period of service of unilateral givers is shorter than it should be.

7. ILLUSTRATION OF AN INTERLOCKING GROUP ORGANIZATION

In an institutional setting one of the male staff smacked a child. There was an administrative outcry, and the man was immediately shifted from the unit. In a mixed group of children, the incident occupied a whole session. The children were indignant about the matter. They wanted me to take sides and express an opinion. Did I agree with children being smacked? I said that I personally did not smack children, but many parents did and felt they were doing the right thing. I asked them what they felt about this, and, to a child, they were against it. Children should never be smacked because it hurt them. I pointed out that this was what the parents intended; but then, one of the children remarked that it was often worse to be scolded. 'That', said another child, 'is only because there is something the matter with our minds: it makes us sensitive.' What she objected to was that the smack had been on the bottom; that was very undignified. 'They think you can treat a child any way you like. Mr P only beat John because he was teasing him about kissing Mrs X.' This was the first hint that the children knew something more than they had previously let out. When asked about the kissing they had supported John because they did not like Mr P.

In the staff group that followed, the members were also highly indignant about the situation, especially because Mr P had been removed. The boy had been asking for it for a long time, they said; he was a real troublemaker; he was not maladjusted; he was just a malingerer. They also tried to induce me to take sides: did I think it was fair that a member of the staff should be removed unheard just because he struck a bad boy for using a very dirty word with regard to Mrs X. When I asked what the word was, Mrs X blushed and said she would rather the matter was forgotten. (The word, I discovered later, was 'prostitute'.)

In a mothers' group shortly after, the mother of the boy said to me: 'I hear he got hit by one of the staff; I can quite understand why; he is really a most provocative boy. Just before he was admitted, I gave him a smack and he said that he would tell his father that he had caught me kissing the milkman. I had to give him half-a-crown even though it was quite untrue. I knew what a suspicious man my husband was. . . !'

So far it appeared therefore:

(1) That the child used the same threat with the nurse, when he got smacked as he did with his mother when he got half-a-crown.

(2) That without seeing any smoke, he had diagnosed a fire and then fabricated the smoke. Was this also true in the case of his mother?

(3) The children had known it to be untrue but wanted to get an unpopular member of the staff into trouble.

In a final mixed group of staff and children some time after the boy admitted to the staff members that he had made up the story and when they asked him why he had done it, he replied: 'It's what I always imagined they were doing. When I first came in here I imagined all the men and women were having sex together and couldn't get it out of my mind. I thought Mrs X shouldn't do that sort of thing because she had children.' This is as good an example of transference in childhood as one could find.

The example illustrates, among other things, how useful a mothers' group can be to complement the groups of the unit, the complex relationship between outside and inside worlds, past and present, adult and child, parent and parent-surrogate. It illustrates the operation of a group technique, the ramifications of a disturbance through a community and its localization in the outside world of one of the children. Finally, it reveals the unconscious knowledge that people in residential establishments accumulate about each other.

The application of analytic group psychotherapy to residential units not served by a staff of qualified therapists naturally raises many questions of theoretical and practical interest.

The technique is directed towards the resolution of interpersonal problems confronting small groups whose composition can be maintained over a certain minimal period of time. The treatment effects may be multiplied by increasing the number of groups to a point at which every individual in the community has been assimilated into one or more of them, and the activities of these small groups can then be coordinated with the wider community programme.

Every sub-group of a residential unit is, to varying degrees, amenable to this line of therapy, but the different systems of relationship (child–child; staff–child; staff–parent; staff–staff; staff–visiting psychiatrists, social workers, or psychologists) would offer different types of difficulty in making groups, maintaining them, and using them to the best therapeutic advantage.

The various groups would be, for the most part, self-governing, although always needing some unobstructive form of 'conducting' or chairmanship. They would be regarded as voluntary associations that had come together willingly for a common therapeutic purpose, and would be kept together by the development of an autonomous group life. The groups would cut across the established hierarchies of a residential community.

The 'key' group, and the one most difficult to run, would undoubtedly be the staff group,which might do a lot better with an outside conductor, say a visiting psychiatrist or P.S.W. This would make for the most economic and effective use of such a person, when he was available.

Because of the 'common denominators' there would be a great deal of mutual influence at work between the groups so that the latent psychological life of the community would gradually become more manifest and disturbance more easily located.

'Levels' of treatment would assume that all sections could do with some of it, but that the intensity would vary with the nature of the group. The children's group would enjoy a full therapeutic experience with the possibility of abreacting both positive and negative feelings. The child's point of view would be presented to other children. In the staff–child groups, the conditions would again be reciprocal, so that the child's point of view would be fully presented to the staff and vice versa. The staff group would understandably have a limited therapeutic purpose, and the word 'treatment' may perhaps be wisely eschewed from its context. Their meetings would focus on special difficulties with children and on difficulties with special children, and the aim, as with other groups, would be not primarily to create insight or explore a deeper motivation, but to undergo, in common with others, a 'corrective emotional experience'.

8. THE GROUP TREATMENT OF PSYCHOTIC CHILDREN

It can be seen from this chapter that the treatment of children of different ages and suffering from different conditions is a logical extension of the group-analytic approach. Its fruitfulness can be enhanced by the concurrent group treatment of different significant individuals in the child's environment. Group therapy of the child with collateral group therapy of the parents is a feasible and effective therapeutic intervention. This has been true even of such unreachable children as those suffering from psychotic autism and symbiosis. Relatively successful groups of this nature have been carried from periods of two to five years in London (Maudsley Hospital) and at the University of North Carolina in the United States. The psychotic child in the group situation is likely to develop panic reactions that lead to further autistic retreat into unreality. As in the 'small room' technique, it is necessary to insist that the child remains with the group and that the room is small enough to resist complete isolation. Nevertheless, the child is allowed periods of regression and withdrawal, when he is left to himself, or actively assisted in regressing to earlier modes of adaptation. At the onset of a panic reaction, resulting from the terrifying closeness of others, a physically restraining contact with the child may help him to endure it. The presence of co-therapists, male and female, their matter-of-fact acceptance of the infantile impulses in the child, and the 'naming' of feelings are also important components of the therapy. In the mothers' group the immense personal dissatisfactions of such women are recapitulated in therapy which comes to mean one further situation in which their needs are unfulfilled. In the fathers' group, it is clear that the child is seen as a rival for the attention of the wife, and, therefore, frustrating to father's dependency needs. On the other hand, it is clear that he also withdraws from his wife's anger and discontent, escaping into a world of his own. It is possible from the three group therapy situations to learn what each member brings into the family environment to produce such a devastating pathology in the child. One gets to know how pathogenic the various members are, and how vulnerable to the influence of one another. A picture of the 'family ego' can be built up on the basis of the different group reactions. It is seen in these cases to be fixated at a fairly infantile level of interaction.

In the children's group, concrete group structures are created by the therapist prior to any psychological group formations as if in anticipation of what is to happen. The motley collection of children, unrealistic and unrelating, are encouraged to act like a group, hold hands like a group, interchange objects like a group, take turns like a group, play games like a group, requiring recognition and reciprocity even though there is a complete absence of real group feeling. The therapist's expectation and anticipation are justified in that the group structures are eventually filled in by genuine group responses and the group begins to behave like a group rather than a collection of automata, and demands group experiences. The retreat into autism is halted and then reversed; strong symbolic relationships appear; and finally, this is followed by the emergence of the individual. It is only when the process of individuation begins that authentic group responses occur. It is still a tenuous and fragile phenomenon; the least excess of pressure drives the patient back into pre-group autism and symbiosis. With a careful dosage of support, stimulation, and sympathy, the psychotic child will venture out into exploratory group interactions, at first only transiently and returning every now and then to his symbiotic shelter for 'emotional refueling' (Mahler). It is a case of two steps forward and one backward most of the time, and if the therapist can tolerate the slow rate of progress, he will arrive one day for a group session and be amazed by what he observes. The development of the group is where most neurotic groups begin but where most psychotic groups end. At this point, it is wise to place the psychotic child in individual therapy.

9. THE GROUP AS A DIAGNOSTIC INSTRUMENT

The psychiatrist, in his diagnostic interview, has the opportunity of seeing two children, the one child looking even physically different from the other – the clinic child and the group child. Unfortunately, he does not always avail himself of the group interview, and may carry away the impression of a pale, sad, inhibited child, looking somewhat 'dead', and with very little to say for himself. Should he, by chance, place the child in a children's group for a period long enough to let him 'warm up' after his clinic experience, he will observe him opening out like a japanese flower in water, suddenly full of colour and spontaneity. A remark often heard in a child guidance clinic is that such-and-such a mother had painted her child as a lion, and when he walked into the clinic, he was just a little lamb. Half an hour in a diagnostic group would convince the psychiatrist that a mother knows a lion when she meets one.

Perhaps the day will come when no child in any clinic anywhere in the world will be placed in psychotherapy without a diagnostic evaluation first in the family group and then in the peer group.

Chapter 9

Group-Analytic Psychodynamics

1. GROUP AND INDIVIDUAL

Group psychotherapy raises many questions. What is the meaning of 'individuality' in the group situation? What forces create and disrupt human relationships and govern the integration and disintegration of groups? What are the most important dynamic processes upon which therapeutic operations depend? Social psychologists have not hitherto provided any theories that do justice to group-analytic experiences and bring order into this field of observation.

Work with therapeutic groups, with people under the pressure of suffering and conflict, gives access to facets of personality and of personal interaction which are deeply hidden and inaccessible in other circumstances. The nature of this material and the group-analyst's familiarity with the language of symptoms, with the unconscious meanings of utterances and reactions, allows him to observe and understand phenomena hitherto concealed. This gives him new insights and reveals new aspects of those sociological groups which have already been studied.

Hence the need for the construction of theories which will penetrate more deeply into the dynamic structure of groups than any which can be formulated through experience with ordinary types of groups.

We know that positive forces of sympathy, love, affinity, liking, interest, and attraction operate in every group as strongly as negative tendencies to hatred, jealousy, rivalry, mistrust, and fear. Wherever human beings meet, even if there are only two of them and they meet for only a short time, they always do react upon one another. It is impossible to imagine that if someone has been alone in a room and a second person enters, the first person will take no notice, or that people stranded in the waiting-room of an isolated station on account of traffic delays or bad weather will not strike up some sort of acquaintance. Whatever refinements may develop in our understanding of group behaviour we cannot doubt that enormously strong forces operate immediately in favour of mutual attraction and mutual reaction between members of any group.

Many years ago the present writer was working in an observation ward for acute psychiatric cases. The patients were only in the ward for a short time and the beds were of an old-fashioned type, rather like cages, so that patients could not leave them, and several yards apart. Yet, every morning a distinctly noticeable mood permeated the ward. This mood manifested itself no matter how mentally isolated the patients were or how different their individual illnesses. Whether this arose in reaction to the matron or ward sister, whose own mood would certainly have a relation to feelings in the ward, or to mutual infection among the patients, the fact remained: on one day everybody was quiet and satisfied, on another everybody was howling or crying or miserable, on a third everybody would be stubbornly silent, and on a fourth talkative.

Even in the most isolated and insulated conditions, in certain kinds of stupor and in catatonic episodes, human beings do retain some relationship with the environment. It is possible to make contact with them and to see them react to certain stimuli in their surroundings, sometimes to a very surprising degree. If these forces compel interaction even in such extreme conditions as these, how much more will they do so among normal or nearly normal people!

The existence of interactive forces in a group is a basic fact which applies also in therapeutic groups. Whatever else we may find in a group, we shall never find that people can ignore the group situation. Man is primarily a social being, a particle of a group. The apparent possibility for him to live as an isolated 'individual' is the result of later, more complex developments. The assumption of a 'social instinct' inside this individual could be looked upon as an example of Freud's concept of the 'conservative' nature of instincts, in the sense that their 'aim' is to restore a previous state of affairs. The more elementary and primitive the level of human existence that we observe, the less personal individuality and independence from the group do we meet. This can be seen even in historical times.

What stands in need of explanation is not the existence of groups but *the existence of individuals.* The phenomenon of an individual standing in relative isolation from the group is something which only began to develop in historical times. We must remember that our species is many millions of years old, so that even the most ancient observations reliably known to us relate only to comparatively very recent times, and even the most primitive communities still in existence are relatively modern products of man's social evolution. We can then gauge how very young, how very superficial, is the development of individuality which begins to emerge in the period of history.

If the emergence of the apparently isolated individual, capable of confronting and reacting to other isolated individuals, belongs to the recent history of our species, we need be less surprised that these individuals react on one another freely in groups of all kinds. It appears that individuals react in the group as if it were their matrix, from which they emerge only slowly, tentatively, and under special conditions. When a number of isolated individuals are brought together, total strangers to one another, there is small cause for wonder that a peculiar struggle of conflicting tendencies arises. In this struggle we can observe bewilderment, suspicion, fear, and impulses to withdraw, and yet, in the face of these, an overwhelmingly strong impulse, amounting to an absolute and irresistible need, to make contact and to re-establish the old and deeply rooted modes of group behaviour. We think indeed that as soon as the group takes hold and the formerly isolated individuals have felt again the compelling currents of ancient tribal feeling, it permeates them to the very core and that all their subsequent interactions are inescapably embedded in this common matrix.

It is this basic conviction that the group is a more fundamental unit than the individual which goes beyond the more usual emphasis on interpersonal relationships and reactions. This refers to the practical conduct of groups as well as to theoretical thinking. In both, the group as a whole is put into the centre. There seems little doubt that future research will establish the adequacy of this hypothesis.

2. THE CENTRAL SIGNIFICANCE OF INTERPERSONAL RELATIONSHIP

Turning from these general considerations to their application in the psychiatric field, attention must be drawn once again to the point that psycho-neurosis is here considered as a disturbance in an individual's relationships. The neurotic person is both more isolated from society and more fixated to a group than normal people. He is more isolated from society than is good for him, than he can tolerate, and at the same time he is more fixated upon his original group, namely the family group.

In a psychotherapeutic group he is therefore torn between the fear and reluctance he feels towards participating in it, and his far more urgent need to be understood by it and related to it.

The character and importance of *relatedness* is therefore seen with special clarity in a group of people with neurotic disturbances, and this may be the reason why its fundamental role is more clearly apparent to us than to those who observe more conventional groups. Relatedness, seen as taking place within a basic all-embracing group matrix, is the corner-stone of our working theory.

The phenomena of relatedness and of disturbed communication, which appear in ordinary life as disturbed behaviour, have another aspect. There are many, very different conditions which concern us as psychiatrists. There are the so-called psycho-neuroses with the manifold clinical pictures they present; psychoses, character disturbances; people who cannot deal with their fellow men and become delinquent or outcast; or people who are not at home, in a sense, with their own bodies; and many other conditions with whose treatment we are concerned. In all of them, without exception, the condition involves the patient's interrelationships, and often the first and most subtle indications of a disturbance are those which appear in relation to his family, his friends, his club-mates, or his colleagues at work. At the same time these relationships represent, at least in sum total, the most powerful reagents in the direction of either cure or breakdown.

The fact that all the disturbances that we ever seek to treat by psychotherapy or group psychotherapy stand out significantly as disturbances in interpersonal relationships cannot be merely peripheral and accidental. This should surely make us think, and should by itself be a strong hint that we are on the track of factors of central importance. Treatment in a therapeutic group can renew the capacity for social relationships and improve it, and can reform and even revolutionize the character of those relationships.

Such changes in the quality of social relationships are of fundamental importance, they affect the innermost core of an individual's personality and in them we have a means of judging and influencing the condition of the patient in its essence. Hence the idea of the group situation as the proper place for therapy, and the conception of the group as a basic matrix whose sinews are interrelationships, interactions, and modes of relatedness, and whose nodal points are its individual members.

3. CONFIGURATION AND LOCATION OF DISTURBANCES

From this fundamental hypothesis regarding the nature of groups we can go on to evolve two other major concepts. The first relates to the *configuration of disturbance* and the second to *communication*, verbal or otherwise.

The illustration which we gave on pp. 110–12 of the pattern of a disturbance involving a daughter and her two parents provides us with a simple model of what is meant by such a configuration. The principle which can be illustrated and supported from observations of therapeutic groups is 'that every single event in a group, even if it seems to involve only one or two members, has a certain configuration which involves the group as a whole'. Such an event is part of a '*Gestalt*' (configuration) of which it is the 'figure' (foreground), whereas the 'ground' (background) is manifested in the rest of the group. It is the same relation as that between the hero and the chorus in the Greek tragedies.

Loss of the leader. Sometimes the group is prominent and the factor which precipitated its reaction is in the background. This can be illustrated by the case of a group which has just lost its leader in the shape of the psychotherapist. It is something which occurs quite often in a hospital, where a doctor often leaves and has to pass on his group to another doctor. In replacing the doctor as the group's conductor we have often had occasion to observe the reactions of a group to this loss, which is felt by it to be a most important one. We have watched these reactions, reactions of annoyance with the old conductor for his desertion, reactions in favour of idealizing and glorifying the new one, or mixed feelings of acceptance and rejection, and we have observed, too, the devious and distorted ways in which all the feelings are expressed (see pp. 88–9). In this case it is easy to see to what event the group is reacting. The *location* of the disturbing factor is known and permits us to distinguish the pattern or configuration of the group's reactions. The cause of the disturbance is the loss of the conductor and the disturbance is configured around the group's relationship to the old conductor and the new one.

In this particular case we are in the fortunate position of knowing quite definitely the precipitating factor, and we are consequently in a much better position to interpret and understand the meaning of the group's reactions even though the individual members of the group may only be vaguely conscious of it, and may talk of seemingly remote and unrelated things. But it is safe to assume that very often in the course of our therapeutic work similar systems of meaning are operative though they may often be unclear to us at the time. Our task is to discover the unknown factor operating behind the behaviour of a group, using as our clues the group's reactions and contributions and our own knowledge of unconscious meanings.

The assumption implied here, if justified, is of considerable theoretical interest. We are saying that the group tends to speak and react to a common theme as if it were a living entity, expressing itself in different ways through various mouths. All contributions are variations on this single theme, even though the group are not consciously aware of that theme and do not know what they are really talking about.

A hospital band. The configuration with which we have chosen to illustrate our proposition, that of the group reacting as it were in unison to a central event or theme, is a relatively simple one. In practice the configurations are usually more complicated. The group often splits up in various ways – sub-groups of members form, and even sub-groups representing only certain aspects of the personality of members. These sub-groups may react at the same time to different things in a competitive way, and we may then see a competition between different themes striving to make themselves heard. There will be an interplay of themes, struggling with and interpenetrating each other. Again, a disturbance in the group may be located in a latent clash between two members over a certain issue. This difference itself may be unknown to either member or to the group, but certain tensions in fact related to it may have become noticeable. A general feeling of tension will probably appear first, followed perhaps by silences, the voicing of discontents, allusions, none of these being clearly understood until gradually, bit by bit, the evidence accumulates and it becomes clear to the conductor and everyone else that the real focus of disturbance lies in the disagreement between these two members. In this case the location of disturbances lies in the disagreement between two members and the repercussions of this are manifested in the conscious and unconscious effects on the whole group. Everyone is drawn into the pattern of disturbance and its resolution equally affects, and gives insight to, all.

This pattern of behaviour is well illustrated in some observations made by the present writer at Northfield Military Neurosis Centre* which we quote here:

. . . the hospital band had been rather sadly failing of late. I went out (it was on a Sunday morning) to one of the huts where the band, or what was left of it, was supposed to practise. It was a dark morning, fairly cold and in the centre of the long hut the band had somehow succeeded in lighting a stove. I found there, sitting round the fire, a pianist, a trumpeter, a violinist, and a drummer, all members of the old band, and another pianist and a clarinettist, who were newcomers to the band.

The group analyst makes contact and observes. I made my contact with them so as to be admitted without disturbing their intimacy. This was easy enough, as I enjoyed listening to their music. It soon became apparent that the two pianists were rather at loggerheads. They were blaming each other for playing *in two different keys.* One of them, whom we will call 'the psychopath' because such was his psychiatric diagnosis, turned out to be a professional musician, a member of a dance band in civil life. He had been the pianist and leader of the previous hospital band. He unceasingly expressed criticism and disapproval of the other pianist, a brave man, not easily discouraged and an ex-prisoner-of-war. The psychopath carped at him for having no sense of rhythm and altogether no idea of playing. He accompanied this by repeating, 'It is not my business as I am going out on Tuesday, but . . .'. The new pianist, his proposed successor, after long and most patient toleration of this consistent provocation, all in the presence of the other members of his band-to-be, controlling his rising temper, finally hit back and declared, 'O.K. then, I am not interested.' At this stage the psychopath seemed satisfied. He went away and returned with another pianist. Meanwhile

* In *Introduction to Group-Analytic Psychotherapy*, Heinemann, 1948.

the drummer, himself a very good musician, who was apparently a faithful pal of the psychopath, mixed in. He had obviously been waiting for a chance to attack the new leader, foreboding a clash of rivalry to come. The tension had been rising continuously up to this point. The psychopath had mentioned already that he was intending to fetch a 'vocalist' – his girl friend. At this point he decided to search for her and they all decided to go back to their wards to have a cup of tea.

Walking back with them towards the hospital, I took occasion to contact the prisoner-of-war, to express my appreciation of his performance and generally to steady and encourage him.

The group analyst acts. After the interval I talked to the men together. I put the cards of my observations on the table and said that it could not have a good effect on their cooperation if their new pianist was discouraged and run down in front of the others. It was quite likely that the old leader, being a professional musician, was more efficient at his piano, but this would be of little help in view of his leaving the hospital on Tuesday. In fact, it was better for him to leave the new band alone. It took some doing, but the effect was that the psychopath left the room, shrugging his shoulders. When he had left, I took the occasion to offer them all help in finding new talent amongst the hospital population. They could, for instance, put up posters in the admission ward and perhaps find some pals in the painting hut to paint these posters for them. In this way I was at the same time promoting the linking up of various groups, all of whom were not functioning too well at that moment, my all-embracing aim in all this being to coordinate and bring to life again the hospital activities. There was a rising spirit of agreement noticeable in all except the drummer, who seemed ambivalent. Now the A.T.S. girl, the vocalist, was defending her friend, the psychopath, from being misunderstood. He was always misunderstood. 'He is really a nice chap if you *know* him.' Others voiced a difficulty: there were plenty of able musicians in the hospital, they said, but they were all afraid to come forth, because they feared if they did well in the band they might lose their chance of being discharged from the Army. I reassured them on this point. (Our policy at this stage of the war was predominantly to rehabilitate people for civilian life and only those who were likely to be fit enough to participate in the Japanese war were to be retained. A large proportion of our patients were, in addition, ex-prisoners-of-war.)

The group carries on. After this the band settled down to practise and the P.O.W. pianist was reinstalled. The newly brought in pianist seemed also ready to participate. His attitude was not quite transparent.

This was the beginning of this band. It started performing during the same week. It found no difficulty in recruiting new members. After a further week or two, it was one of the highlights of the hospital. No 'social' in the club was conceivable without it, and there was one nearly every other night. It also settled its problems of suitable accommodation for practising and the like. They played very well indeed. After a few weeks the band, now composed of quite different members again, was unaware that I had ever had anything to do with its existence.

Oedipus Tyrannus. The process we have described may also be reversed, and a disagreement between two people may turn out to be the expression of two conflicting tendencies in the group, which has been personified and voiced as it were by these two people.

We see this process at work in the theatre where characters in a play not only speak as individuals but can express a conflict of feeling present in the audience as individuals and as a group. An illuminating illustration of this was presented in a contribution to the *Psycho-Analytic Quarterly* some years ago in an analysis of Sophocles's play *Oedipus Tyrannus,** though with no conscious reference to group psychotherapy on the part of the authors. The hero of the play, King Oedipus, has killed his father Laius and has married his mother, Jocasta. Oedipus does not know that the man he killed was his father, nor that Jocasta is his mother. Nevertheless the city of Thebes, of which he is now king, is struck by plague, and the oracle declares that the disaster is a divine punishment which will continue until the evil-doer is discovered and punished. Oedipus has committed 'the only two crimes which troubled primitive society'† patricide and incest. He therefore stands in the play as the representative of the wish in Everyman to commit these crimes, and must in turn be punished to assuage the feelings of guilt in Everyman which the active presence of these wishes has aroused. The tragedy presents a conflict of wishes in the mind of the audience, the wish to commit Oedipus's crime and the wish to escape its consequences. The character of Oedipus stands for the one wish and the chorus for the other, and the tragedy is played out between them. The authors of the article write '... the tragedy gives us an excellent opportunity to study the reactions of a community towards a hero who has violated taboos, but has gained a position which makes him its protector. The negative attitudes are not manifested as open hostility to the hero; they are nevertheless as clearly expressed by the tendency of the chorus to

* Joel Friedman and Sylvia Gassel: 'The Chorus in Sophocles's *Oedipus Tyrannus*', *Psycho-Analytic Quarterly*, vol. XIX, no. 2, New York, 1950.

† Freud: *Totem and Taboo*, 1913.

remain objective. The chorus does not become actively involved in Oedipus's travails, nor does it exert itself to prevent him from going to his doom. By remaining detached, it absolves itself from responsibility . . . actually the chorus maintains a driving demand upon the hero to fulfil what the community expects.'

The chorus expects Oedipus to find the murderer (himself) and 'Oedipus accepts fully the responsibility which the community is so eager for him to assume. . . . The chorus is not unlike a helpless community which is in the habit of throwing responsibility to the leader (father). . . . At each point it is called upon to make an active decision, it retreats into a state of helplessness and suffering which serves to reinforce its demands upon Oedipus.' Eventually Oedipus discovers that he himself is the criminal and accepts punishment. 'Once the hero is put out of the way, the chorus is in a position to evaluate its feelings; it can view life from a new perspective that moves to higher standards. This ability to utilize the experiences of the hero for its betterment and wisdom is directly connected with its psychological need to have the hero removed.'

We have thought it worth while to spend some time on this illustration because it demonstrated so many of the mechanisms we see at work in the therapeutic group: the inescapable emotional tie uniting actors and audience,* between members who are active in the group at any moment, and those who are passive; how the conflicting tendencies in the group find their spokesmen who voice feelings common to all; the group's defensive mechanisms, which operate to preserve its ignorance of its own wishes, and to project them on to an individual scapegoat, very often the conductor, who is the person called upon to 'know' the things which the group does not yet dare to know; how the re-enactment of the drama of a conflict under the guidance of the conductor can lead to a re-evaluation and re-integration of feelings which finally make his presence unnecessary; how the chorus as opposed to the hero, the group as opposed to the conductor or any one member, becomes the field in which the basic conflict is located.

* In this context we would like to acknowledge the particular debt which we owe to the work of J. L. Moreno. In his system the insight into the dramatic situation is basic, and he uses dramatic techniques as the main vehicle of psychotherapy. Moreno's so-called psycho-dramatic and socio-dramatic techniques and his theoretical concepts have also become significant in the field of group psychotherapy, and are in accord with many viewpoints expressed in this book.

4. COMMUNICATION AND THE THERAPEUTIC PROCESS

So we come back to the basic theoretical assumption that any event in a group must be looked at as something which potentially involves the whole group although it may be expressed in endlessly varying configurations. Symptoms which are located physically in a single individual, so-called 'conversions', correspondingly appear in the group only negatively as areas of 'no response' so long as their meaning cannot be expressed in words.

This leads to the concept of *communication.* Group-analytic theory has long recognized communication as a process of fundamental importance in group behaviour and in psychotherapy. A study group working in the framework of the International Congress on Mental Health held in London in 1948, and of which both the present authors were members, took communication as its main object.* The view of communication taken was a comprehensive one, and it was considered as a dynamic process.

In the United States a school of thought has developed which presents communication as the basic concept for the whole of psychiatry (viz. Ruesch and Bateson: *Communication: the Social Matrix of Psychiatry*).

We are all familiar with the ordinary processes of communication, which we use daily to make known our thoughts, feelings, and needs to others, and by which we can in turn understand the thoughts, feelings, and needs of others. Such communication takes place on a conscious level and is in one way the equivalent of the manifest occupation of a group which we discussed earlier. (See pp. 33–4.)

But just as we distinguished a group's occupation from its preoccupation, so in the case of communication we wish to draw attention both to the many additional meanings which can be conveyed in the process of communicating a message with a simple definite content, and to the many ways in which we are all continually communicating impressions to one another in a sense unintentionally. For example a stranger may ask us the way to

* ***Report of the Preparatory Commission dealing with Communication, particularly Verbal Communication, with Reference to Group Analysis.*** **Prepared for the International Congress on Mental Health, London, 1948.**

Piccadilly Circus, communicating quite clearly his need for information. At the same time he tells us that he is a stranger at least in that part of London, and he may also tell us by his accent and the inflexions of his voice that he is a Scotsman, that he is worried or late, that he is shy or self-confident, and perhaps something of his position in society. Or again we may sit opposite someone in the train who never speaks at all, and yet by his dress and posture, by the colour of his skin, by his fidgeting, his tenseness, or his repose, he may communicate much to us which we can register in our minds and understand. Then there is that sort of communication which takes place between players in a football game who respond and react to their colleagues and opponents in a pattern which has meaning for all.

In talking of communication we are thinking of all these processes, conscious and unconscious, intentional and unintentional, understood and not understood, which operate between people in a group. At one end of the scale are deliberate verbal communications fully understood and responded to, and at the other, symptoms and inarticulate movements. Between these two extremes lie all those modes of expression which are steps in a ladder mounting from one extreme to the other.

Anything that can at all be observed, or perceived, or reacted to in a group is potentially a communication. At the same time, as Ruesch and Bateson point out, no process has fully become a communication until there are signs that it has in fact been reacted to, that it has linked a transmitter and a receiver. The process need not be conscious, but it probably is partly conscious as soon as it deserves the name of communication.

We have described earlier how, as soon as a group is formed, there is an inevitable interaction between members and a need is felt among them to make more and more contact, to establish more and more common ground, to enlarge their understanding of others and to be better understood themselves. These forces all operate towards establishing communication, which in its turn opens up new pathways of contact and new areas of understanding. Communication in a very real sense *is* this process.

The fundamental instrument of communication is language, and language is itself born from the need to communicate, from that very force which impels the members of a group to interact. When we select language rather than action as our chosen instrument of therapy in the group we are choosing the most perfect instrument of communication which the group possesses. At the same time it is an instrument not finally forged and shaped, but one which has shared a common history with the group, and shares also its common future. It is an instrument forever on the anvil, continually under the hammer of new experience and feeling arising in the individual and the group.

Because words are old and so carry layers of meaning and because they must be spoken by individuals who attach meanings to them which are private as well as public, and because they are called upon to reflect internal and external events which are always partly new, their common meaning in a group has always to be re-established, and a gap always exists between what they mean to the user and what they mean to the hearers. This semantic problem, set by the nature of language, is of great importance in therapeutic groups. It is important as a method of education but also as a process in itself.

When we discussed symptoms we discovered that they were both the expression of a conflict and an attempt to conceal it. A symptom is thus a compromise formation, a compromise between the need to express something which could be understood by all and a need to suppress such expressions by reticence, disguise, and distortion. As therapists we enter this struggle between the patient's need to become conscious of his underlying conflict, to face it and to tolerate its being known to others, and his need to keep it hidden. When the problem is conscious, it can be clearly communicated and understood. The patient's struggle takes place in the sphere of communication and has to be fought out there if therapy is to be effective. It is for this reason that the therapist must be an expert at *translation*, so that he can at the right time help his patient in this fight.

Part of therapy consists in bringing this struggle to an issue, and we have already gone a long way towards a solution – in fact we have opened the way to a complete solution – as soon as the mental problem which underlies the symptom can be expressed in words and discussed. A conflict consciously understood and formulated faces us like a territory mapped. We do not alter the territory, but we can now choose a route; we cannot avoid the hazards of life there, but we can arm against them, we know what we have to fear and in knowing this we set bounds to fear itself.

Group Psychotherapy

Once a problem is conscious, communicated, and shared, we can enlist the help and experience of others in its solution. For example it is impossible for the other members of a group to make anything of one member's headaches. But if and when the headaches have at last been translated and expressed as a conflict in this person, which may be between his wish to lead a happy life with his wife and his anger at her inability to give him the foremost place in her affections and put him before her mother, this problem can be communicated, understood, and shared by others.

The process by which a patient passes from developing headaches to a consciousness of his mental conflict, which can be communicated, is a long and difficult one. This process in a group is related to and possibly identical with the process of making the unconscious conscious that forms the basis of psychoanalytic treatment. It is closely related to *verbalization* for, as Freud showed, unconscious thoughts attain to consciousness by becoming attached to verbal representations.

We can see then that to become conscious, to verbalize, and to communicate are integral parts of the therapeutic process. It is extremely probable that we are describing a single process, or at least various aspects and stages of a single process in using any of these terms. In a group-analytic group the force which drives members of the group to interact and communicate is encouraged and cultivated. In such a group therefore we find considerable pressure in favour of communication, in favour of understanding and being understood, in favour of increased consciousness, articulateness, and verbalization. Under this pressure and with the therapist's encouragement and skill as a translator, the inarticulate, unsharable, autistic symptoms of patients are gradually reshaped in the continual process of communication as ever more articulate formulations of problems. This process, as it unfolds, can be studied in all its variety at many levels and throws light on the essential dynamics of psychotherapy in any situation.

It is hoped that this discussion has to some extent clarified what we mean by saying that communication is a process which moves from remote and primitive levels of the psyche to ever richer and more articulate modes of conscious expression, and that it is closely bound up with the therapeutic process. This is a most important concept for group psychotherapy, for psychotherapy as a whole, and for the study of communication, particularly verbal communication, whether in its conscious or unconscious significance.

The three basic concepts which we have now outlined – concerning the essential relatedness of individuals in a group, concerning the location or configuration of disturbance, and concerning the nature of communication – are closely interrelated and express aspects of group behaviour as a whole. Group relationships could not exist or be made visible without communication, and disturbances could not be located. At the same time if there were no essential relatedness between members of a group there would be no communication and no location of disturbance. However, if we remember that the term communication can mean both a channel or path, that is a structure, and also an active process, that of making common, and if we think of it as including both these meanings, then it can be said that communication is the overriding concept of the three. Perhaps we can see in the close linguistic affinity between the words 'communication' and 'community' an unconscious recognition of this fact.

We have had occasion to indicate earlier how the phenomena observed in individual psychoanalytic treatment appear also in group treatment. A list of some equivalents was given in Chapter 3 (see p. 52). For example, when a member of a group voices a fact in so many words, in such a way that other members of the group can understand it, this is equivalent to the individual patient becoming conscious of some hitherto unconscious content of his psyche in psychoanalysis. The group equivalent for the process of repression, denial, splitting, and so on could also be shown.*

5. SPHERES OF RELATIONSHIPS

There are also other aspects of psychological relationship, which are of basic theoretical importance for the study and treatment of groups and we should like here to touch on some of the ways in

* See S. H. Foulkes: 'Group-Analytic Dynamics with Special Reference to Psychoanalytic Concepts', *International Journal of Group Psychotherapy*, vol. 7, 1957.

which a group and its members can be significant to one another. We find the formulations made by Wernicke* and E. H. Erikson† particularly well suited to the material we have observed. Erikson distinguishes three spheres of relationship between an individual and his social and material environment, which he relates to stages in the development of the child. There are firstly relationships in an *autocosmos*. In the autocosmos we experience and know only our own body and its states, and we experience other things only in terms of the body. Secondly there are relationships in the *microsphere*. In the microsphere the child knows and understands objects beyond his body, but he knows them mainly in terms of his own phantasy and wishes. He endows objects with qualities projected from his own mind, the sofa becomes a boat, the doll an angry mother, the mother a witch, as the need arises. Thirdly, there are relationships in the *macrosphere*, in a world genuinely shared with others in which a horse can only be a horse and a table is an object with qualities in its own right, qualities arrived at by the sharing of observation and experience between individuals.

These spheres of relationship, in terms of which the child experiences his environment as he grows up, do not disappear and vanish but continue to operate in the mind, integrated under the primacy of thought in the macrosphere. The first two modes of experience reassert themselves whenever integration is imperfect and colour mature thought in the macrosphere. In psychoanalysis the effects of more primitive modes of relationship can be observed and identified in the transference, and they can also be observed in the group.

Much more could be said about psychic functioning in each of these spheres, particularly as it is seen in individual psychoanalysis. However, we wish to confine ourselves to phenomena which can be observed in the group situation, and will only refer here to Wernicke's observations on psychotic patients which serve to amplify Erikson's description of autocosmic behaviour. Psychotic thinking operates in terms of the autocosmos, and Wernicke noted that his psychotic patients tended to refer their disturbances sometimes to events occurring within their own minds, sometimes to events occurring in their own bodies, and sometimes to events occurring in the external world. He described these three systems

* Carl Wernicke: *Grundrisse der Psychiatrie*, Leipzig, 1906.
† Erik H. Erikson: *Childhood and Society*, Imago, 1951.

of reference as auto-psychic, somato-psychic, and allo-psychic. Thus although in the autocosmos experience is apprehended in terms of the body and its feelings, this does not mean that only the body is apprehended. Even in the autocosmos there is relationship, and even relationships at this level can be reflected in the group situation.

Relationships in terms of the autocosmos operate at a very deep level in the mind and a group can seldom become conscious of them. In the group-analytic situation it can be seen that individual members do experience sometimes other members, sometimes the whole group, as projections of their body or mind image.

Relationships in terms of the microsphere certainly do manifest themselves in the group. This is the sphere, *par excellence*, of transference relationships. The group can come to represent, in the minds of its members, the community as a whole or social conscience, and an individual will feel ashamed, embarrassed, or rejected if the group judges him. Not only can the conductor in his person come to represent these things but the whole group can do so. Furthermore the conductor and the group can also come to represent the objects of what is called object relationship in the maturer macrosphere, for example husbands, wives, and friends. Their feelings towards such people, or rather towards their inner images of such people, can be projected in the group. At one moment the conductor may be seen as an almost god-like idealized parent, at another as a bad parent who is feared and rejected, or the group as a whole can be treated as a mother, or individuals in the group can react to one another in terms of transference in a stricter sense as if to their sisters, brothers, mothers, husbands, or wives.

In this connexion the interesting observation can be made that, in certain respects, a patient's transference relationship to another member of the group can be a more intimate one than the original relationship itself. In one group a man and a woman were exchanging information about their respective marital problems and it became clear that a transference relationship existed between them. Each stood for the other's partner in marriage and both were raising questions which each would really have liked to discuss and clarify with his or her spouse. After both had been made conscious of this significance of the situation, neither felt that it would be possible to speak at home as they had in the group.

Matters which each found too intimate to discuss with his or her respective husband and wife were not too intimate to discuss with one another in the presence of the group although each was and remained fundamentally a complete stranger to the other as a private person.

These levels of relationship, which we have been discussing, all operate in the group and may all operate at the same time, or the group may operate first on one level and then on another.

All concepts used in discussing group behaviour should be concepts specifically derived from the study of groups. The application of ready-made concepts from individual psychotherapy only serves to blur the sharpness of our observation and distort it, whereas the study of groups will help us to understand the phenomena in both situations more clearly. In the complicated multi-dimensional network of group relationships we cannot keep track of events if we try to see them as a mosaic of individual interactions. We observe a total process, and it is to this total process that our therapeutic levers must be applied. Theoretical concepts which are needed for the very practical purpose of handling this intricate process should be formulated in terms of what we can actually observe.

Chapter 10

Wider Theoretical Formulations and Applications

1. GROUP AND COMMUNICATION

Group-analysis used as an instrument of treatment, teaching, and research has a bearing on all human activities and experiences. It raises problems about, and may offer solutions of interest to, philosophy, semantics, psychology, psychoanalysis, education, art, religion, and social and cultural movements and organizations. It opens the gates towards a new social psychopathology and a dynamic science of psychotherapy. What follows are theoretical formulations arising from group-analytic observations and speculations as to their significance.

Communication and reality. As the process of communication has been found important, let us begin with this. How does the group help us to know about the world, its reality, and the relationship of this to mental reality, unconscious phantasy, and the possibility of communicating about these? Our immediate guarantee for an object's existence is our perceiving it. Its existence *is* its being perceived, as Berkeley put it. On the other hand we feel quite rightly that what we perceive is not of our making, that there is something independent, a world of 'objects' by virtue of which we can have perceptions at all.

Thus the 'subjective' and 'objective' aspect of experience gives rise to a philosophical dilemma. It seems to me that it is precisely group observation that can help us here. Let us take a concrete example. Suppose we are talking about the city of Paris: this is a place which may be beautiful, which lies on the Seine, where one can eat, drink, walk about, take a taxi. . . . And we do not doubt that even if we have ceased to exist, this Paris will still be there. It may be experienced in a more personal form; perhaps as the town where I missed my train, or where I fell in love, or saw a good ballet; as a town that I like or dislike; a town which today may be far away, but tomorrow may be on my way, and very near in my mental scheme. There is then not *one* Paris, but many thousands of 'Paris' which all exist in equal reality. For every thousand of observers there are as many thousands of 'Paris'. Yet all of them relate to some *one* thing which is in existence, and to which all observers react, as distinct from a hallucination which has no existence apart from its only perceiver. How then do we form the notion of independent reality? This Paris which does exist is a commonly held idea or concept of a place, which emerges from the interplay of all the individual experiences of Paris. Human beings are mentally sufficiently near to one another, have enough ground in common to understand each other's experiences and to communicate them to other people by the use of words. With the help of words we can thus make statements about a Paris that does exist independently of any of us individually.

Suppose we let a hundred people pass through a room, one at a time, and ask each one independently (assuming they were all English-speaking people), 'What is that?' and pointed to a chair, they would presumably all say without a doubt: 'That is a chair.' There must therefore be something characteristic in this particular piece of furniture, something which resides really in the object, and not in the beholder, which enables all to call this object by the noun 'chair'. Our experience of that particular chair in that particular room would have a hard core of common ground and differ only at the fringes. So firm is the core in this case that language itself could not be violated without casting doubts on the observer's sanity – as for instance if one of them were to call the chair a 'horse'.

While recognizing this independent objective world we must not overlook however that we are in a large measure interested in things in so far as they affect us. This shows itself in the connotation of the words we use, because various concrete and well defined 'objects' have for us humans some special significance. To us 'the sky' means something high, something in which the sun, moon, stars move, from which sunshine and rains come. 'The sea' is a moving volume of water, rivers flow into it, one may swim, one may drown in it, one may be in a boat or in a large ship travelling overseas. We need only think of what the 'same' sea may mean to a fish, or to another water animal, or the 'sky' to a bird, to see how very differently – if they could speak – their linguistic categories would have to be constructed. The world reflects the beholder. We are interested parties. Disinterested comment on the world around us is the aim of scientific investigation. But where our interests are involved, human experience is not just suffered, rather is it an active selective process related to what we want and what we can in fact achieve. For this reason our statements about objects do often reveal something about ourselves as well, in a quite personal sense.

Social model of consciousness and the 'model of three'. Wherever any kind of experience exists, there must be *at least two agents reacting upon each other*: two systems must meet, come together, and in some way, one might say, must even clash. Perhaps some degree of conflict, though not necessarily in the psychoanalytic sense of the word, must exist between two systems in order to constitute the possibility of an experience. (*Objectum*, object, *Gegenstand*, express standing in opposition.) Is it possible that consciousness itself rests on the same fundamental condition? For a species of beings to develop consciousness it might be a necessary precondition that its individual organisms (nervous system) can behold at least two different items at one and the same time. This condition is certainly fulfilled in us individually, and a competitive situation inside the psyche would bring consciousness into operation.

Relativity of truth in the interactional field. In our groups, human beings meet and interact not with lifeless objects but with other human beings. To establish a consensus in such a situation might be thought an insuperable task. While it is relatively simple for individuals to agree that a chair is a chair, it is much more difficult for them to agree for example about the quality of A's attitude to B.

A states: 'B is angry and feels angry with C.' In making a statement about an event between B and C, A can make observations in relation to B or C without himself being B or C, and furthermore can focus upon the relationship itself from outside in a way which B and C, being actively engaged in it, cannot Three people are included in the statement. This configuration – which I have called 'the model of three' – is the simplest model of group interaction.

Very much more complex interactions occur in a small group of six or eight members. If we consider that, in our groups, verbal communication, that is words and sentences, predominates, and that these words may have completely different connotations for the people concerned, how can we really assume any sort of understanding to take place?

Yet such understanding is in fact progressively established. The group does not get more and more confused but more and more clear about the significance of A's words and sentences. On account of this empirical observation that understanding is progressively established in a group, the following working hypothesis has been found reliable: observations such as 'B is very angry with C tonight' may be treated as if they were elementary perceptions. We accept such statements as simple, factual, and elementary. They are no more and no less astonishing than the notion, 'that chair is green', or 'this shoe is brown'.

At the same time, if A says 'B is angry with C', we assume, as in everyday life, that he means by 'angry' what we also mean by 'angry'. We find that we can operate with this word and that a process goes on by which we gradually arrive at an understanding about the word 'angry'. As to the statement itself, we need not assume that it is true in an absolute and objective sense, but rather that we have to investigate into the sense in which it is true, where it belongs so to speak. What is really going on can only be elucidated on the basis of what has been stated in A's, B's, C's, and my own terms.

As we know, it may well be that B was not angry with C, but A angry with C when he made his statement. We may therefore get a statement by B: 'Not at all, I am not angry with C.' Or we may get a statement by C: 'I thought last time you were angry with me, as a matter of fact, but I did not feel you were so now.' After some analysis the question may be raised whether A himself is not in fact angry, and he may in turn reveal that he had observed certain reactions of B to C which he did not like, and that he may have been slightly jealous, etc.

Thus, by an analysis of all these aspects we arrive at a total picture of what was going on in the given situation when A said B was angry with C. There may, in the end, be several different statements according to whether events are seen through A's, B's, C's, or our eyes, and yet *they are all valid* in that they now each make sense from everyone's point of view. We thus arrive at a common ground of understanding which allows at the same time for the difference in meaning for each person. We need not assume that there is only one real and true account of what has happened, and that what we hear are more or less subjectively coloured and distorted versions of it. Instead we assume that all these statements are true in a *relative* sense; there are as many part-truths as there are observers – indeed as no participant can be in the selfsame position as any other, their accounts must differ at least slightly. Thus we extend the relativity theory into the psychological, interpersonal, field.

On the basis of our premises we can accept all contributions as valid communications. This is the necessary and inevitable counterpart of the concept and technique of 'free group association'. The group is bound to establish a common language by which the range of its direct communication is constantly enlarged and qualitatively more precisely defined. We have said that such communication is necessary if any therapy is to take place, and that it is closely linked with the therapeutic process itself. We now take a step of great consequence in submitting all communications to the processes of *interpretation*. This is concerned with *meaning* – the most complete and precise meaning we can obtain – both as to content and interaction. Content refers to verbal as much as to any form of non-verbal expression; interaction refers to persons as well as to mental processes. The corresponding operations applied to the manifest material, the observable data, are in the first place: *translation* (deciphering) and *location*. The process called location is the mapping out of disturbances, behaviour, and other events in the 'matrix', by which we mean the dynamically interrelated network, the psychic fabric of the total group.

Thus the interpretation of any statement or behaviour presupposes that it is first of all observed and accepted as a communication, that is to say as something addressed to someone else (a message) and something which at least potentially can be understood. This message is then processed by the operations of translation and location. It may then simply be 'received', or else in some way responded to. The process of analysis comprises this response in addition to the interpretations of the situation in the sense just described. In addition to receiving the message, the analyst may make his interpretation or part aspects of it explicit (interpret in the usual sense), he may comment on the message, confirm or contradict it, link it up with other observations, point out contradictions or demonstrate these by confrontation, and so forth. In the therapeutic group the process of analysis takes place with the active participation of its members.

In this analytic procedure we observe the following principles concerning communications:

(1) That we consider all communications as relevant, the actual completed communications as well as the intended ones, the manifest as well as the latent and unconscious ones, the verbal as well as the non-verbal communications.

(2) That we take equally into account all other responses and reactions, thus promoting them to the rank of communication, as it were.

(3) That every event in a group is considered as having its meaning within the total communicational network – the matrix – of the group, though often more particularly relating to one or several of the members. This constitutes a 'figure-ground' relationship within the group.

We will now take another example. A says: 'Have you heard this voice calling? I heard someone calling me "Take care, or else he will poison you!"' This is what in general psychiatric jargon is called a delusion: A has heard a voice. Again we do not argue this fact with A; we accept that a voice has spoken to him. If in fact the voice were a delusion, an hallucination or illusion in A's mind, and had no existence beyond A's mind, how would this tell in the group? First of all, all the others will say that they have not heard the voice. Indeed they would probably be immediately aware that A was deluded and say 'you're barmy', or 'you must hear voices', or 'you must be deluded'. This makes it clear that the voice is confined to A – a significant observation. Our next step is to see what A does with this experience, how he reacts to it. He may do all sorts of things. He may insist that the voice was real, and perhaps construct some theory to explain why the others did not hear the voice; he might say that it is clear to him that although everybody heard the voice, they are pretending they did not because they are all in league with the person who is going to poison him. That is, he will show what is called a paranoid reaction.

We would conclude: 'Well, A heard this voice and has an incorrigible conviction that it is real. He behaves in such a way that he cannot accept the fact that no one else heard the voice as evidence in this matter. Indeed he at once invents an explanation for their failure to hear it.' Assuming now that we wait for the group's reactions, it might happen that Y says: 'Of course there is no such voice as he says, but I did really one day think "I wish I could poison him".'

This is somewhat oversimplifying what may happen, but it will illustrate the point that even a delusional statement is not necessarily confined entirely within the mental area of one person, but has a certain relationship to the others. It may be that in a much more subtle form the idea of poisoning was in the group's mind, perhaps in the shape of destructive oral phantasies directed symbolically towards A or towards other members of the group. We find even in such an extreme case as this that there is, somewhere, 'a grain of truth', that there is somewhere a corresponding complementary factor to which the individual relates.

Paranoid ideas in a group serve to indicate the presence of hidden undercurrents and wishes in the group or in individual members, such hidden wishes providing the 'grains of truth' to which the ideas relate. These paranoid interpretations of patients relate directly to the *unconscious* attitudes of other people, and this is where psychological gift and paranoid disposition come close together. One can envisage a paradoxical situation arising in which two patients, or a patient and a therapist, might each attack the other's interpretation as paranoid. This relative truth of paranoid interpretations can present a real difficulty which has to be overcome and which often presents a most intractable problem, since paranoid structure is very hard to modify, not least because it is a normal mode of ego-functioning as well as a manifestation of mental disturbance in certain cases.

I think it would be possible to show, on a very deep level, the essential superiority of the group situation for handling this problem. In the group, as opposed to the individual situation, many opinions are forthcoming when such an impasse occurs, some taking one side, some another, and some remaining intermediary. There are many witnesses and their testimony provides a fuller context in which to evaluate the pattern of events. The question as to whether the paranoid formation yields to group treatment is a matter of considerable practical and theoretical interest. One group under supervision, composed experimentally of selected paranoid patient, stackled this problem and the results were promising.

It is certainly clinically true, as I have mentioned, that these paranoid and other psychotic responses which come up occasionally are extremely useful and valid indications of hidden currents in the group, and can function as a kind of psychological seismograph.

2. THE TRANSPERSONAL NETWORK OR MATRIX

At the centre of all our thinking about communication in groups is the concept of the group network or group matrix, which we have touched on earlier. The group is a matrix of interpersonal relationships, and the events which occur in it are interpersonal phenomena. These relationships and these events exist literally in between two and more people; they do not occur in one person or in another, but can only come into existence through the interaction of two or more people. We have here a new element under observation.

Attention in the past has been focused on illness as a function of the individual personality, but all illness ('mental' and 'physical') and every disturbance involves social relationships. Very often the earliest signs of change for better or worse show themselves in interaction with others.

The social matrix can be thought of as a network in quite the same way as the brain is a network of fibres and cells which together form a complex unit. In this group network all processes take place, and in it they can be defined with regard to their meaning, their extension in time and space, and their intensity. Their definition within the network of the group matrix we have called their *location*.

J. Ruesch and G. Bateson have developed similar concepts in their work and speak of the 'cultural network', of 'intrapersonal communication', and of 'interpersonal communication' in the group. Our own type of group work offers quite unique opportunities for the study of the process of communication in a multidimensional sense.

The group matrix can be regarded as the operational basis of all mental processes in the group in the same way as the individual's 'mind' is the operational basis of all mental processes in the individual. Its lines of force may be conceived as passing right through the individual members and may therefore be called a *transpersonal network*, comparable to a magnetic field. The individual is thought of as a nodal point in this network, as suspended in it.

Particularly through their nervous systems and brains the organisms of the group members are in a state of interaction, in a common field, in interpenetration and communication. They speak now through one mouth, now through another. Active currents within the group may be expressed or come to a head in one particular person, between particular persons, or may, in a sense, be 'personified' in individuals. But whatever is going on in the group is always regarded by us as a process developing in the total group.

Communication is everything happening in this particular group situation which can be noticed, it is everything sent out and received with response whether consciously or unconsciously. Such communication involves many levels of the mind at the same time, and has meaning on all of these. At any given moment the level on which the communication is mainly operative will depend on the sender and the receiver.

In thinking of mental levels we may picture them schematically as steps on a staircase. Below a certain step on the staircase the mental content is, as a rule, 'unconscious' in the analytic sense, and is expressed in 'primary' language. Only under certain conditions does such content mount into the upper strata and become conscious. On the top level of the staircase is clear, logical communication in words. At this level the 'secondary' processes of the mind operate, secondary in the psychoanalytic sense in contrast to the primary processes of unconscious thought. Words are the chief vehicle for the communication of articulate (secondary) thought, but it is the process of communication itself which specially interests us, not the factual transmission of information through words.

When the level of complete communication has been reached, nothing further can be done with the particular problem involved, except to solve it if it is not already solved when reaching that level. But the neurotic disturbance – not to mention the psychotic one – is bound up with deficient communicability and is therefore blocked. It has no access to the free, undisturbed communication of higher levels. The language of the symptom, although already a form of communication, is autistic. It mumbles to itself secretly, hoping to be overheard; its equivalent meaning conveyed in words is social. This process of communication is the medium of all other therapeutic agencies. It drives the therapeutic process forward and enables the cathexes and conflicts, the difficulties and agglutinations in lower levels of the mind to be surmounted. Thus there is a move from symptom to problem, from dream to the conflict underlying the dream. This is certainly one direction in which the process of communication operates towards expression in ordinary language.

3. MODEL OF DIFFERENT LEVELS OF COMMUNICATION

In order to make certain points of interest more intelligible, let me use a purely schematic diagram as a model (see Fig. 13). The zero or base line we will assume to demarcate roughly the frontier between what is normally conscious and what is normally unconscious. Above this line are all the modes of communication which are used manifestly under normal circumstances. They are shown on an ascending scale. We will quite arbitrarily assume six degrees (lines) above zero, and call them positive (+), and six below, which we shall call negative (–).

Only the middle six degrees, from +3 to −3, are concerned with words and correspond to verbal expression or communication. Degrees from −4 to −6 correspond to bodily equivalents of emotions, organ language, conversions, and structural changes. From +4 to +6 correspond to abstract symbolic languages, for example to mathematics, pictorial symbolisms, and probably also artistic communications in painting, music, etc., although the latter have peculiar qualities, since their span comprises the whole scale, while jumping so to speak over the verbal sphere.

The ascending scale might range from ordinary conversations (= +1) to more and more abstract concept formations. Capacity to use abstract symbols corresponds to a greater capacity for differentiation.

The descending scale corresponds to primitive modes of expression, e.g. through the body. If verbal or thought material is concerned this is subject to the primary process. It is primitive thinking, pre-logical, as released in psychotic thought or action. This is unconscious in the psychoanalytic systematic sense (belonging to the system *ucs*), on our table symbolized by × in contrast to conscious thought, belonging to the system *cs*, which is marked O.

Our schematic notation will thus look as follows:

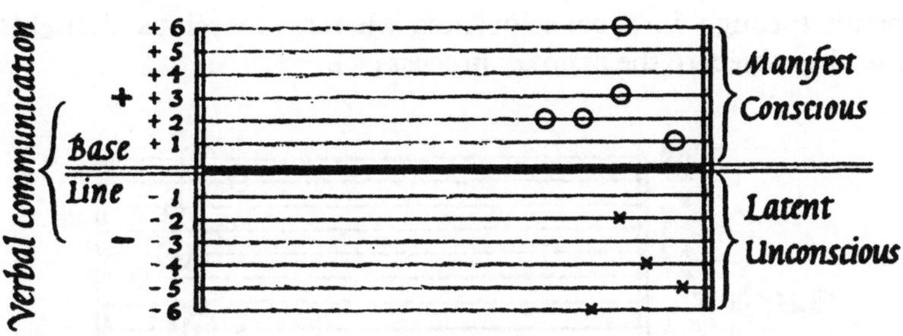

Fig. 13

× = ucs (primary process)
O = cs (secondary process)

Under usual circumstances, all *ucs* formation (×) would be latent, unconscious, and would not interfere unduly with the *cs* formation (O) above the zero line. We indicate this schematically on the right of our Figure 13.

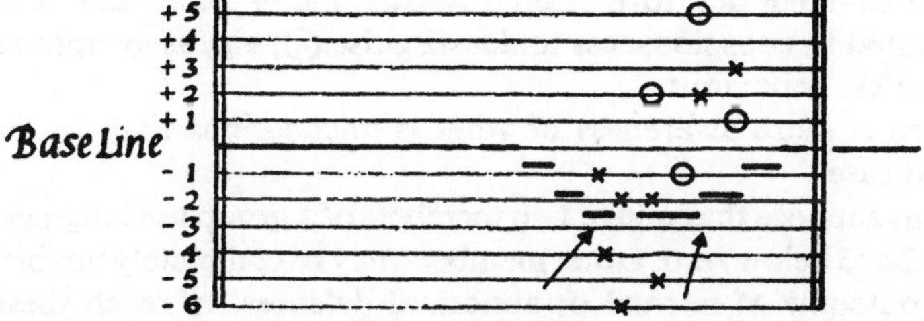

Fig. 14 [*Psychotic*] × = ucs O = cs

All sorts of mental conditions presenting characteristic features can be shown schematically on the diagram. For the sake of illustration only, I will present in Figure 14 and Figure 15 a psychotic and a neurotic picture respectively without, however, enlarging upon them here.

This schematic picture of psychotic illness shows much of what would normally be below zero appearing in consciousness. The borderline between conscious and unconscious is disrupted and lowered towards the negative side. Arrows indicate the pressure of unconscious formations towards manifest expression – in the last resort towards ego involvements and action. *Ucs* elements break through into consciousness whereas conscious thoughts may be subject to the primary process (×).

Fig. 15 [*Neurotic*] × = ucs O = cs

In the neurotic picture the base line is not fundamentally moved, but has gaps. However the base line is also hardened and reinforced (repression, reaction formation). There is some pressure of overcharged *ucs* formation towards the + side and it is manifested in consciousness under disguise ⊗, e.g. as symptoms in manifest behaviour.

There is more awareness of what is unconscious than in the normal case.

Let us suppose that one or two members of a group use language round 2 or 3 below zero. Other members may be completely unable, as an outcome of normal or abnormal defences, to reach these levels, to understand what is being said. The therapist's aim is to reach down to 2 or 3 below zero for these two, to see how far up they can go, and at the same time to broaden and deepen the expressive range of the other members, to increase their understanding of the deeper unconscious levels.

The aim is to establish, as soon as it can be done, a communal zone of understanding. In this particular example it may extend from −2 to +2 on the diagram. This would be the area of communication in which the group can move. Anything can now be taken up, as far down as -2 and as high up as $+2$. There is always, to be sure, an *unçonscious understanding* present upon which we build up.

The general tendency will be for the level of the group as a whole to rise until the shared zone of communication can include the top level of ordinary conversation ($+3$). Thus this part of the process is fundamentally akin to education. The understanding and expression of the group as a whole is guided and brought up to a higher level. At the same time the equally important process of deepening understanding takes place. The group has to go downwards and to deepen its understanding of the lower levels of the mind by broadening and deepening its vocabulary until every group member also understands these levels. Ideally the whole group should learn eventually to move over the full range of our scale.

Moving the group's level of communication upwards corresponds to progress in maturation. In learning to communicate, the group can be compared with a child learning to speak. If the child is too readily understood by its parents on an infantile level it will make no effort to increase its mastery of language.

A rising level of communication in the group is not to be confused with intellectualizing. Intellectualized discussion is suspended, as it were, in mid-air, whereas true communication in the group is firmly rooted in the experience of the group, and grows from it.

Mental conditions vary in their severity, which can also be expressed by the degree of deviation, qualitatively and quantitatively, from the usual distribution on this scale. What range in their severity can be usefully brought together in one group may be gauged by the ground it can cover as regards communication. If individuals are mentally so far apart that they cannot meet at all, or only with great difficulty, then they are not suited for the same group.

4. SOME EQUIVALENTS OF PSYCHOANALYTIC PROCESSES

There are, I think, in the group, *equivalents* of processes which are known to us from psychoanalysis. However, it is interesting to think of them in a different way, namely, as taking place in the group as a whole, in the group network, rather than as taking place within the intra-psychological field of each individual.

We may begin with the concept of *group consciousness*. We have already mentioned that we can follow Freud's meta-psychological formulations regarding the connexion between consciousness and word representation. Thus we can say that what is conscious – in the group – is what is actually voiced by somebody. Something said and heard, and understood by all, would be completely 'conscious'.

The 'preconscious' may be exactly represented by anything which *could* be voiced and understood by all, but does not happen to be. The group cannot of course talk about everything, and there are innumerable things which could be stated in the group, but which do not happen to be stated. These would be the preconscious ideas.

'Unconscious' would be those thoughts which are present in one or more members, but which these members feel prevented from voicing and so bringing to the attention of all.

These models exactly correspond to the psychoanalytic conscious, preconscious, and dynamic (or repressed) unconscious. We may ask what would be the equivalent of 'repression' in the group model. It would be, for example, if something were not being voiced, were not in a state to be voiced, because everyone was afraid of thinking or saying it, or because there were apprehensions about it in view of the presence or the expressed attitude of certain people.

We can see quite easily on this model that mechanisms operate similar to those described by Freud. Certain things which ought to be expressible cannot be and are not voiced because of other forces active in the group, which are stronger and more highly charged (reaction formation).

A 'denial' comes about in a similar way, and can be represented in the group model. Something which concerns the group or the group members may be hotly denied, ignored, or passed over.

Mechanisms of 'splitting', 'reaction formation', and 'dramatization' can equally be represented in a group model. There is also a group equivalent of 'symbolization'. Somebody may, for instance, symbolize the conscience of the group (super-ego), or its impulsive wishes, the *enfant terrible* (the id), etc. This is to mention only a few such mechanisms, in particular defence mechanisms. My point is to show the principle of thinking in group models, models really belonging to the group.

Memory in the group. Another type of example is the following, which may throw light on the development of 'memory', or 'recall'. It is often interesting to observe when and how the group reaches a stage at which somebody can refer back to a previous event, at which somebody asks 'do you remember . . .?', thus appealing to the group's memory of past events. This has some relationship to the type of group (open, closed, etc.). It is fascinating to watch the beginning of memory, the operation of memory, the appeal of memory; when, how, by whom, and at what stage it is possible to invoke it; what are the minimum preconditions, the distance necessary for the event to be experienced as a memory.

Every group, especially a closed one, will bring up remarks such as 'do you remember last time somebody asked so-and-so?', 'you remember you were annoyed with me about such-and-such': these things are not felt as a memory, we are still in them. What I mean by memory is a reference to things fully past, as when a member says 'I still remember – I don't know if anyone else does – how when you first came you said X was a very fine fellow, that you admired him. . . .'

One may say that memory is after all the property of an individual mind or brain mechanism, and that this is a rather unnecessary translation of it into the group model. I am not sure about this. I have sometimes felt, although I have not so far made any systematic study of it, that actually it is just the other way about: that we really have used such observations which come from our social 'togetherness' and our experience in the social situation to illustrate what goes on in our minds or brains.

In this connexion we may remember that Freud talked of 'the censor', taking as his model, quite deliberately, the function of an outside, political censor. Or again, when he described 'the repressed' how he said that the repressed was not allowed into the room of consciousness, that there was a doorkeeper.

Such illustrations as these show, I hope, not only how a function of the mind like memory can be seen to operate as a function of the group network, but also how the group lends itself to the study of processes which have hitherto been regarded as internal psychological processes of the individual mind.

5. DIFFERENT THERAPEUTIC GROUP SITUATIONS

In situ. Group-analytic psychotherapy and group-analytic research branch out from the kind of therapeutic group we have made the centre of our present study into many related spheres. They can be applied *in situ*, of which the band group we described (pp. 238–41) is an example, that is in the group where a disturbance actually arises, such as the family, the sports team, the factory cadre which we go into the field to investigate. These are the groups in which a patient's disturbance is now expressed, not where it belongs genetically, but where it belongs in the living present.

Root group. Alternatively we may make the actual members of the disturbed field of interaction the objects of therapy in our consulting room. I propose to refer to this type of group as a 'root group' (R-group) in order to indicate that the disturbing conflagration roots in this group, at least in the present. Usually, of course, the conflict is a transferred one from the original root group, genetically, as a rule, the family. Sometimes the primary genetic root group and the actual, present one are identical. Treatment in the 'root group' is as yet being practised only on a small scale and experimentally, but with much promise. These types of group stand in contrast to the treatment group we have described, which are 'transference groups' (T-groups), where every member is a potential auxiliary ego and a focus of projection, and where every relationship can be a model by proxy of relationships in society outside. Transference and projection operate of course in every type of group, but in these treatment groups they are thrown into relief.

Our concept of illness as a function of relationship necessitates the recognition of the principle of *ramification*, that every illness occurs in a nexus of relationships in ordinary life. Logically, our technique of treatment should accept this and be ready to take into the therapeutic setting all persons who prove to have a therapeutically relevant relationship with the patient, but practical obstacles are as yet considerable.

In a 'root group' type of treatment our patient might be a

married man and we might then be led to include his wife in the treatment. We might presently find that a friend of the wife's was deeply involved and later that the husband's stepmother also played an important role. Our idea would be to trace and to accept the ramifications of the disturbance as far as they are operationally relevant and to enlarge our group to include all these people either simultaneously or in various constellations and different settings.

The group-analytic group. We have long advocated the possibilities of the group situation and, in particular, the therapeutic group (T-group) situation as a method of study for all sorts of problems. The studies made at Chestnut Lodge by Stanton and Schwartz* are highly interesting examples of this approach in the clinical hospital field, as also were those made in the therapeutic community at Northfield. The ideas developed at Northfield have since been rediscovered and applied (though only partially) at various places, but do not seem to have been grasped or carried out as fully as they were in the original experiment.

The group can be made the basic medium of therapy. This idea has been put into operation at the Out-Patient Psychotherapy Department at the Maudsley Hospital, London.† Patients are received in a preliminary group. They then join a preparatory group before they may become members of various special groups. Treatment begun in a proxy (T) group might be continued in a root (R) group or in an *in situ* group, or in an individual situation with the therapist, or vice versa.

Proxy groups. In a flight of fantasy I have even considered that under circumstances it might be useful to reconstruct actual interpersonal situations entirely by proxy. Suppose, for example we had a number of patients who were interrelated, and each of whom was being treated in an individual situation by a different therapist. Let us assume, for instance, that one therapist treats the father of a family, a second his wife, a third their daughter, and a fourth a close friend, each patient being in individual psycho-

* A. H. Stanton and M. Schwartz: *The Mental Hospital: A study of institutional participation in psychiatric illness and treatment*, Tavistock Publications, 1954.

† S. H. Foulkes and A. Parkin: 'Out-Patient Psychotherapy: A contribution towards a new approach', *International Journal of Social Psychiatry*, vol. 3, pp. 44–8, 1957.

analytic treatment. In such a case it might be highly interesting for the therapists concerned to see the problems of these individuals in a common perspective. It would be undesirable to disturb the isolation of each individual therapeutic situation, but they could be brought together through a meeting of the therapists. At this meeting each therapist could represent his patient, each being 'briefed' through his knowledge of his own patient's reactions to the others, and together the therapists could reproduce the original social situation by proxy in dramatic form.

Social therapy. It can be envisaged that the group technique will eventually involve (in therapy) the whole community and bring together everybody concerned in a problem, not only doctor and patient. In short, it will bring neurosis back where it really belongs, for such problems are problems which concern the whole community, as we can see, in the case of delinquency or other social and psychological difficulties which afflict our society.

The application of group techniques can take an infinite variety of forms, varying in emphasis and intensity and stressing as more useful either the analytic or the occupational side. Ultimately, these techniques raise the whole question of social therapy on an even larger scale. Our concern is with the development of techniques, and of ever more appropriate situations; with their application and interaction; with the way problems are expressed and constellated in them; with the effect of these techniques on each other; and with the possibilities of each as a method of exploring areas of behaviour yet uncharted.

Study in action. In conclusion I should like to return to some considerations regarding theory. Psychoanalysis was, historically, largely based on the assumption that we are dealing with conditions which have a definite cause and point of origin, a time at which they arose, and which also have a diagnosis, a prognosis, and a cure. Lately psychoanalysis has made a strong move in another direction, towards a study of the dynamic relationship between the therapist and the patient as the centre of the therapeutic process. With this we are in sympathy.

In our conception of psychotherapy we find it less important to discover and diagnose the history of a case than to study how an illness presents itself currently, and how, in what direction, and by what means we can hope to change its course. The concepts with which we operate (our emphasis is on the *operational process*) deal with insight, capacity for insight, cooperation, attitude. These, as we know from our daily practice, are the important things *in fact* for what we do. They govern our decisions as to what we can and ought to do, our views on the prospects for each case and how we shall try to treat it.

Our need is for a dynamic science of psychotherapy, which uses operational concepts and which is studied, formulated, and applied in the actual process of therapy. It will study the processes of change through clinical observation in the therapeutic situation, fully accepting and exploiting the idea that therapy is research and that research in this field is therapy.

Objections are raised to psychoanalytic and psychotherapeutic observations on the grounds that they are necessarily subjective and imprecise. Such demands for a 'precise science' collecting data amenable to exact measurement and statistical manipulation are based on outworn physical concepts of the nineteenth century, which have been superseded in our field of study, notwithstanding the great value they may have for the investigation of material to which they can appropriately be applied. This is made abundantly clear in the various studies of communication to which we have had occasion to refer. Our immediate clinical observations are the fundamental elements from which we start. They are observations that can only be made in the interaction of therapist and patient, or in the therapeutic group situation in which the therapist participates. Nevertheless we emphasize that they are elementary observations from which to start.

We submit these observations to group investigation. Thus we apply to them the very test and process which decides what is true or false, right or wrong from the point of view of human beings. To what degree values are relative or universal also establishes itself through their operation in the group, as does the individual's mode of deviation in respect of these values.

I should like to illustrate this point once more by a simple example.

A therapeutic group is observed by three observers apart from the conductor. One of these is Mrs A. All observers are agreed that in this particular session the men discussed manifestly the question of marrying, but underlying this was their fear of women, and that the women in the group were rather reluctant to talk, and appeared subdued. The one woman observer, Mrs A, adds her particular view, namely: 'The women were afraid of Bob S.' Now instead of asking whether this observation is correct, and if so whether other explanations of the women's behaviour were incorrect, we would rather put it in the following way: what is exactly the meaning of Mrs A's statement? Not, 'is it true or untrue?', but 'on what particular aspect does it throw light?' For instance it might be merely her personal reaction, that she overemphasizes this aspect for reasons of her own, or that she identifies as a woman with the other women in the group and therefore sees an aspect of the truth, which the other male observers had overlooked. To decide on this would need a further analysis with all those concerned, and this is exactly what happens in therapeutic group-analysis.

For interest's sake, some points which have a bearing on our present example may, however, be mentioned.

(1) Bob S has frightened the group earlier on, especially when in an outburst of temper he smashed a window-pane.

(2) At least one of the women in the group has expressed her fear of him, so had the therapist for that matter.

(3) The conductor in his report of this particular session (which had been dictated prior to Mrs A's remark) stated: 'The discussion at this stage tended to remain largely in the men's camp until Bob S pointed out that the married women ought to have something to contribute, at which stage Mrs F said . . .'.

The point here is that it was Bob S who turned to the women and encouraged their participation in this way, possibly indicating some feeling that he himself was inhibiting them. As a matter of fact the interpretation of Mrs A was not in this case at all difficult to reconcile with what the other observers had already stated.

The concepts which we form as a result of such study in action correspond to a new insight into the nature of human motivation, and of human action and interaction.

Selected Reading

ABERCROMBIE, M. L. J. *The Anatomy of Judgement.* London, Hutchinson, 1960; Penguin Books, 1969.

ABERCROMBIE, M. L. J. *Aims and Techniques of Group Teaching.* London, Soc. for Research into Higher Education Monograph, 1970.

ABSE, D. W. *Clinical Notes on Group Analytic Psychotherapy.* Charlottesville, The University Press of Virginia; Bristol, John Wright and Sons Ltd (*In preparation*).

BACH, G. R. *Intensive Group Psychotherapy.* New York, Ronald Press, 1954.

BARNES, E. (Ed.) *Psychosocial Nursing.* Contributions by T. F. Main and others. London, Tavistock, 1968.

BATTEGAY, R. *Der Mensch in der Gruppe.* 3 vols. Bern, Huber, 1967–69.

BION, W. R. *Experiences in Groups.* London, Tavistock Publications, 1961.

BURROW, T. *Preconscious Foundations of Human Experience.* New York, Basic Books, 1964.

CARTWRIGHT, P., and ZANDER, A. (Ed.) *Group Dynamics.* London, Tavistock Publications, 1954.

CASSON, F. R. C. *It's Healthy to be Human.* Revised edn. London, Allen & Unwin, 1967.

CLARK, D. H. *Administrative Therapy.* London, Tavistock Publications, 1964.

CORSINI, R. J. *Methods of Group Psychotherapy.* New York, McGraw Hill, 1957.

DE MARÉ, P. B. *Perspectives in Group Psychotherapy.* London, Allen & Unwin, 1972.

DURKIN, H. E. *The Group in Depth.* New York, International Universities Press, 1964.

EHRENWALD, J. *Neurosis in the Family and Patterns of Psychological Defence.* New York, Harper & Row, 1963.

ELIAS, N. *Über den Prozess der Zivilisation.* 2 vols. Basel, Verlag Haus zum Falken, 1939.

Selected Reading

ELIAS, N., and STOTSON, J. L. *The Established and the Outsider.* London, Cass, 1965.

ERIKSON, E. H. *Childhood and Society.* London, Imago, 1951; Penguin Books, 1965.

FLUGEL, J. C. *Man, Morals and Society.* Harmondsworth, Penguin Books, 1962.

FOULKES, S. H. *Introduction to Group-Analytic Psychotherapy.* London, Heinemann, 1948.

FOULKES, S. H. *Therapeutic Group Analysis.* London, Allen & Unwin, 1964.

FOULKES, S. H., and PRINCE, G. S. (Eds.) *Psychiatry in a Changing Society.* London, Tavistock Publications, 1969.

FREUD, S. *Group Psychology and the Analysis of the Ego.* Standard Edition, vol. 18. London, Hogarth Press, 1955.

FREUD, S. *The Psychopathology of Everyday Life.* Standard Edition, vol. 6. London, Hogarth Press, 1960.

GROTJAHN, M. *Psychoanalysis and the Family Neurosis.* New York, Norton, 1960.

GROTJAHN, M. *The Voice of the Symbol.* Los Angeles, Mara Books 1971.

HEIGL-EVERS, A. (Ed.) *Psychoanalyse und Gruppe.* Göttingen, Vandenhoek & Ruprecht, 1971.

JONES, MAXWELL. *Social Psychiatry in Practice.* Harmondsworth, Penguin Books, 1968.

KADIS, A. L., KRASNER, J. D., WINICK, C., and FOULKES, S. H. *A Practicum of Group Psychotherapy.* New York, Harper & Row, 1963.

KAPLAN, H. I., and SADDOCK, B. J. *Comprehensive Group Psychotherapy.* Baltimore, Williams & Wilkins, 1971.

LAING, R. D., and ESTERSON, A. *Sanity, Madness and the Family.* London, Tavistock Publications, 1964. Penguin Books, 1970.

LEWIN, K. *Field Theory in Social Science.* Ed. D. Cartwright. New York, Harper Bros., 1951.

MORENO, J. L. *Sociometry, Experimental Method and Science of Society.* N. Beacon, N.Y., Beacon House, 1951.

MORRIS, D. *The Human Zoo.* London, Jonathan Cape, 1969.

MULLAN, H., and SANGIULIANO, I. *The Therapist's Contribution* to *the Treatment Process.* Springfield, Ill., Thomas, 1964.

OTTAWAY, A. K. C. *Learning through the Group Process.* London, Routledge & Kegan Paul, 1966.

POWDERMAKER, F. B., FRANK, J. D., *et al. Group Psychotherapy.* Cambridge, Mass., Harvard University Press, 1953.

ROSENBAUM, M., and BERGER, M. (Eds.) *Group Psychotherapy and*

Group Function. Selected Readings. New York, Basic Books, 1963.

RUESCH, J., and BATESON, G. *Communication; the Social Matrix of Psychiatry*. New York, Norton, 1951.

SCHEIDLINGER, S. *Psychoanalysis and Group Behaviour*. New York, Norton, 1952.

SCHILDER, P. *Psychoanalysis; Man and Society*. New York, Norton, 1951.

SCHILDER, P. *Psychotherapy*. New York, Norton (Revised Edition), 1951.

SCHNEIDER, P.-B. (Ed.) *Pratique de la psychothérapie de groupe*. Florence, Ed. Universitaria Barbèra. Vol. I 1965, Vol. II 1968. Vol. III 1972.

SIGRELL, B. *Group Psychotherapy*. Stockholm, Almquist & Wiskell, 1968.

SLAVSON, S. R. *An Introduction to Group Therapy*. New York, Commonwealth Fund, 1943.

SLAVSON, S. R. *A Textbook in Analytic Group Psychotherapy*. New York, International Universities Press, 1964.

SPEERS, R. W., and LANSING, C. *Group Therapy in Childhood Psychosis*. Chapel Hill, University of North Carolina Press, and London, Oxford Press, 1965.

SPOTNITZ, H. *The Couch and the Circle*. New York, Knopf, 1961.

SUTHERLAND, J. D. (Ed.) *Towards Community Mental Health*. London, Tavistock Publications, 1971.

TAYLOR, F. K. *The Analysis of Therapeutic Groups*. London, Oxford University Press, 1961.

THOMPSON, S., and KAHN, J. H. *The Group Process as a Helping Technique*. Oxford, Pergamon, 1970.

WAELDER, R. *Basic Theory of Psychoanalysis*. New York, International Universities Press, 1960.

WALTON, H. (Ed.) *Small Group Psychotherapy*. Harmondsworth, Penguins Books, 1971.

WHITAKER, D. S., and LIEBERMAN, M. A. *Psychotherapy through the Group Process*. New York, Atherton Press, 1964.

WOLF, A., and SCHWARTZ, E. K. *Psychoanalysis in Groups*. New York, Grune & Stratton, 1962.

YALOM, I. D. *The Theory and Practice of Group Psychotherapy*. New Basic Books, 1970.

The following journals have special reference to group and community psychotherapy:

Dynamische Psychiatrie. Editor: Gunter Ammon. Pinel-Publikationen, Berlin.

Selected Reading

Group Analysis: International Panel and Correspondence. Editor: S. H. Foulkes. The Trust for Group Analysis, London.

Group Process. Editor: Max Rosenbaum. The Association for Group Psychotherapy and Process, New York.

International Journal of Group Psychotherapy. Editor: S. Scheidlinger. American Group Psychotherapy Association, New York.

International Journal of Social Psychiatry. Editors: J. Bierer and M. K. Opler. Avenue Publishing Co., London.

Small Group Behaviour. Editor: Wm Fawcett Hill. Sage Publications, Beverly Hills, California.

Index

Index

Index

Index

For Product Safety Concerns and Information please contact our EU representative GPSR@taylorandfrancis.com Taylor & Francis Verlag GmbH, Kaufingerstraße 24, 80331 München, Germany

Batch number: 10725893

Printed by Printforce, the Netherlands